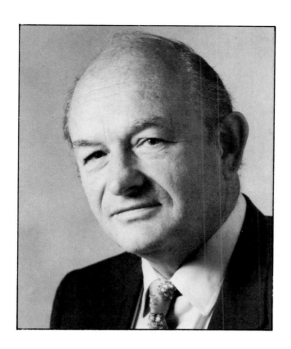

Dr Keith Thompson has had a distinguished medical career and is known throughout the world for his special interest in the care of the aged in the community. His work has been recognized by travelling fellowships and the awards of the Butterworth Gold Medal, and the Gold Medal of the Hunterian Society. He continues to practise as a family doctor, so maintaining constant contact with the elderly community he serves. He has lectured widely, and has appeared both on radio and television. He has written numerous scientific papers, and several books, including *Geriatrics and the General Practitioner Team, Health for Old Age*, and *The Care of the Elderly in General Practice*. He is editor of the journal *Geriatric Medicine*.

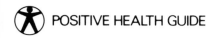 POSITIVE HEALTH GUIDE

CARING FOR
AN ELDERLY RELATIVE
A guide to home care

Dr M. Keith Thompson
MB, ChB, DRCOG, FRCGP

Published in association with
HELP THE AGED

MARTIN DUNITZ

To Chantal and Alex

First published in the United Kingdom in 1986
by Martin Dunitz Limited, 154 Camden High Street,
London NW1 0NE

British Library Cataloguing in Publication Data

Thompson, M. Keith
   Caring for an elderly relative.—(Positive health guide)
   1. Aged—Great Britain—Care and hygiene
   I. Title II. Series
   362.6'0941   HV1481.G5

ISBN 0-906348-93-5

Phototypeset in Garamond by BookEns, Saffron Walden, Essex
Printed by Toppan Printing Company (S) Pte Ltd, Singapore

*A portion of the profits
from this book is donated to
Help the Aged*

CONTENTS

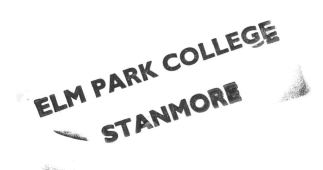

1 UNDERSTANDING AGING

Whatever the reasons for deciding to care for your elderly relative at home, you probably feel daunted by problems that will crop up in the future. However fond you may be of your relative, whether parent, sister, brother, uncle or aunt, there are sometimes going to be heavy responsibilities and social pressures. How will you cope when your relative becomes ill, immobile, incontinent? What will happen if you yourself are ill and unable to care for the older person? How will your relationship survive the pressure of living under one roof after years of independence of each other?

We hope that by explaining the nature of aging and giving some guidance on preparing a comfortable home, you can make your relative welcome and enjoy having him with you, rather than think of your new role as a burden. You should find that by reducing the organizational problems to a minimum, and involving your relative in the day to day running of the house, the emotional problems will often take care of themselves.

So frequently, as in a marriage, it is the tiny habits that annoy. Living together can work successfully only when people have a deep mutual love and are prepared to be tolerant of each other. We hope the practical advice in later chapters will help this harmonious relationship be more easily achieved.

Nevertheless we have to understand what the process of aging is and how it feels to start losing some of the faculties we have always taken for granted. You need some understanding of how your relative views himself or herself as physical and mental changes become more obvious, and how changes in the outside world may affect and disturb someone with less acute faculties.

What is it like to be old?

To each of us, aging is a slow process that passes unnoticed, yet others who observe us after an interval see differences very clearly. The time when anyone thinks old age has arrived will alter entirely from one person to the next. People who have led an active life continue to think of themselves as vigorous individuals rather than old people well into their eighties, while some who retire at sixty or before believe themselves old just because they have joined the pensioner class.

People often think of getting old as a wearing out process, with their bodies likened to a machine. This is only partly true: machines cannot repair or regulate themselves. But we certainly notice we have decreasing amounts of energy over long periods and cannot undertake such a wide range of activities as before. These changes take place slowly, and so we are given ample time to adjust. We can therefore go along happily without noticing much change until a challenge is thrown down. An old sportsman will shout instructions to players on the field, thinking he can demonstrate the right techniques, and will be surprised when he can't run as he used to. Put to the test this way, the deficiencies of age reveal themselves. But it is only when they are constantly shown up that we become depressed about it.

Some old people overrate themselves, thinking they can do as much as they did twenty years ago, but I suspect there are more who have been persuaded to undervalue their capabilities. Probably more harm is done to old people by overprotection than by urging them on to do more. Environment is therefore very important. In agricultural areas and Third World communities old people continue to play a part, though to a lesser degree. The generation gap has developed in Western societies during the last two generations so that old people often do not have a role. This applies both to old men and women, who may feel that they have to appear young, and even enter into competition with the young. Tensions develop, and much more stress is placed on the fact of age.

Surely what is desirable is to feel comfortable with our age and not to become caricatures of either age or youth! Certainly, by closing our eyes we can never get back any idea of our age at a particular time. Usually we feel much younger than we are and the sense of getting old is imposed on us by outside influences.

Attitudes to aging vary enormously. Little children, for instance, seem to be indifferent to age changes, but young people at the height of their physical strength and beauty are often very fearful and resentful of them. Some old people themselves have attitudes that have been formed and conditioned by earlier expectations. Their unfounded worries can have a damaging effect, as the story of one of my patients illustrates.

When she was seventy-nine, Mrs Jones began to decline very mysteriously. Nothing seemed to have changed, and I could find nothing in my examination to account for her increasing weakness, so I asked my hospital colleagues to admit her for diagnostic tests. They were extremely thorough and every possible test was done and found to be normal. Mrs Jones was sent home, and I went to see her, intending to spend half an hour with her. During this time, she told me that she had been influenced as a young girl by some rhyming couplets which hung in a frame on the wall of her home, describing the various ages of man and woman. Of these she could remember only what it said about the woman of eighty. It read:

> Glued to her chair by weight of years,
> She sits and waits till Death appears.

This is exactly what Mrs Jones was doing, and when I explained to her how wrong this old-fashioned idea was, she recovered completely, as mysteriously as she had become ill. Mrs Jones wrote to me when she was eighty-seven, and in good health, to remind me of that visit.

It is important to have positive healthy attitudes to aging, not to blame it for every bad event in later life, and to picture it not as a process of inevitable decline, but rather as a phase of life when we continue to develop. Undoubtedly we alter with age, and much of our behaviour at this time will result from our earlier life. Many people want to compensate for things they missed out on when they were young, such as travel or going to shows; others who have lived a fulfilled life become concerned with their mental or spiritual development. Yet others seem to be little altered in their attitudes and feelings.

So although old people often look similar to each other, with their small stature, whitened hair and glasses, it is vital that we not only recognize their individuality, but seek to retain and develop it. It is easy to wonder who you are, and become bewildered in old age, when you have no job and few family contacts. You can quickly feel yourself a non-person in a strange environment, being called 'granny' and dressed in clothes provided by a charity.

Changes in thinking and behaviour

What are the worries that older people have about themselves and when do they become noticeable? Apart from the tendency to forget names after the age of forty, most of us notice little change in our mental performance until well after middle age – that is, roughly after sixty-five. An old person may be slower in the way he or she responds to questions and become more rigid in adhering to routines in daily life. Her thoughts may be tinged with pessimism rather than optimism, and she becomes more inward looking. You may find these qualities rather trying unless you consider how fixed routines are useful to those with failing mental powers, who do not have new ambitions for themselves.

This confining of behaviour also explains character changes which make old people 'difficult'. By concentrating on essentials and trusted guidelines, a person's character seems to intensify with age. What may formerly have been admirable as a way of life, such as thrift in a housewife, may lead in old age to miserliness. An old man whose earlier success in life resulted from a sense of order and authority may turn into a family despot. Other old people fade or mellow, losing the adult qualities of independence.

Intellectual capacity, on the other hand, may continue to grow. If you think of a crystal growing in a concentrated solution you may picture what happens. While older people lose the faculty of fluid thinking and the ability to manage new concepts, they can continue to build on the structure developed during their lifetime, and there are many examples of remarkable achievements of this kind in old age. The one I like is the way Grandma Moses switched from doing intricate embroidery, when her fingers became too stiff, to oil painting, achieving worldwide recognition. The process of learning for old people is, of course, slower and less complete than in young people. But it is important that mental activity should not stop or be taken over by a helper. It has been shown that assisting old people with tasks actually hinders them, while they do well if they are encouraged to do as much as they can on their own.

What are the needs of the old?

Most of their daily needs are the same as ours, but the elderly do have their particular requirements too, which demand our special consideration. The desire for good food, suitable clothing, warmth, financial security, self-respect, affection and an occasional luxury are universal. While these may be taken for granted by most of us, many old people lack one or more, or even all these basic needs. Anyone caring for an elderly person can see that the list is also incomplete, for there is a need for conversation and to exchange ideas. Too often elderly people spend the greater part of their lives without being able to talk to anyone about their concerns. They need a chance to communicate as much as we do. Old age can and should be a period when there can be development. Of course, your relative's aims will be different from your own – such as career, marriage, and having children – and they will be shorter-term. But it is likely that you will have to spend time planning a realistic programme with your relative.

Where possible, the activities should involve constructive skills and problem solving, and a contribution to the needs of the whole household. Although better than sitting and staring blankly into space, being given childish games does not enhance the dignity of age. To provide creative leisure and satisfaction means thinking about what motivates your relative and demands as well an effort of imagination on your part.

While thinking about the needs of our elderly relatives we have to re-examine the mistaken ideas and prejudices that have grown up about old age. It is extremely difficult for an old person to convince us otherwise when certain attitudes are taken for granted by society. Such attitudes are beginning to change, but too many of us have a poor understanding of the abilities and needs of the older generation.

Why ideas are changing

Before 1950 there were comparatively few studies on aging and old people. Since then there has been one of the greatest knowledge explosions in this field so that even those with a specialized interest have difficulty in keeping abreast. It is important for all of us to have a broad idea of the changes in the aging population. In our interdependent society no one is isolated from the older generation, and eventually most people find themselves caring one way or another for older people, with an increasing proportion looking after their relatives at home.

Everybody knows that the populations of developed countries have aged during this century. What is not always realized is that the proportion of those aged sixty-five will not increase greatly, but there will be a lot more people over seventy-five. We can see this quite clearly in the table below.

The main reasons why so many of us now survive into old age are better nutrition, better housing and better education, which have brought improved long-term health and more successful treatment of disease.

	Total birth-rate* millions	%	Over 65 millions	%	Over 70 millions	%	Over 80 millions	%
World								
1900	1668		c. 50	3				
1980	4432	29	260	5.6	158.3	3.6	35	0.8
2000 (projected)	6119		400	6.5	252.3	4.1	60	1
2101 (projected)	10529							
United Kingdom								
1900	36		1.7	5				
1980	55.9	13	8.2	14.7	5.4	9.7	1.4	2.5
2000 (projected)	55.2		7.7	14	6	10.9	1.8	3.3
France								
1900	38.3		3.3	8.6				
1980	53.6	15	7.5	14	5.1	9.5	1.4	2.6
2000 (projected)	56.2		8.1	14.4	5.6	10	1.5	2.7
United States								
1900	98.8		3.1	4.1				
1980	223.2	15	25	11.2	15.6	7	4.4	2
2000 (projected)	263.8		32	12.1	20.6	7.8	5.8	2.2
India								
1980	684.5	35		3	11.1	1.6	2	0.3
2000 (projected)	960.6				22.4	2.3	3.6	0.4
Japan								
1980	116.6	19		9	6.4	5.5	1.5	1.3
2000 (projected)	129.3				11.9	9.2	3	2.3

*Birth-rate = births per 1000 population

When we look to the future we must be realistic. Some optimists believe that the elixir of eternal life is not far off being discovered, and so there will be an increase in the active human lifespan. The pessimists see in the greater numbers of the very old a tremendous burden of physical and mental dependency and suffering, which will impose an intolerable strain on the sufferers, their families and the resources of the health and social services. Between these extremes lies a third, more probable, outcome. The lifespan of the human race, which has remained fixed for thousands of generations, is likely to remain unchanged (although life expectation, which depends on the environment, has been raised). But the effects of health education, which are already being felt, will delay even further the onset of the diseases of aging. Not smoking, extreme moderation in the use of alcohol, prudent eating, sufficient exercise, the control of blood pressure and a retained sense of social involvement and prestige should contribute to a future when years of pain and infirmity or, if you prefer, early death, could be eliminated. After a full and vigorous life we should simply become frail and enjoy a mercifully short final illness.

For the present this remains no more than a fervent hope. For the forseeable future there will be large numbers of elderly people needing care. This increasingly is being provided outside hospitals, old people's homes and other institutions by relatives, friends and neighbours, for the most part untrained and unskilled. There are all kinds of reasons why people want to look after their elderly relatives, but broadly we could categorize them into:

1. A sense of loyalty and affection, and a wish to repay a parent's kindness
2. The acknowledged need of the older relative for help
3. The undesirability of institutions for the elderly
4. Economic reasons.

Within these broad categories cold duty, warm desire to return affection, pity, respect or sometimes possessiveness – or a mixture of any or all of these – can play a part. When we decide to bring an elderly relative into our home it is important to examine all these feelings and try to get a perspective on how to cope with the emotional strains that are sure to arise. We shall discuss this in more detail in Chapter 2.

What level of care do the elderly need?
Attitudes towards activity and fitness have changed vastly over the last two decades. Yet there is still a tendency to treat all old people as decrepit because of their looks, despite the fact that many still feel fit and active. Fitness at any age depends entirely on the individual and when looking after elderly people we have to decide which activities they want to undertake and would be appropriate for them.

12

It is interesting to compare the way different nationalities think of fitness. Americans are more likely to go to their doctor for poor health but are less willing to accept the limitations of aging than Europeans. The British are twice as likely as either Danes or Americans to say their health is good, even if they are housebound! Whether it is our perception of an elderly person's fitness or that person's own estimation of what can be done, we are learning a lot more from these recent studies that can be applied to the lifestyles of the elderly.

Of course, much of the evidence about the activities of the elderly has been conflicting, and it needs intelligent interpretation. For instance, watching television appears to decrease with age and to be replaced by increased attention to radio programmes. But this must be considered against the background of a generation who spent up to three-quarters of their life with radio as the mass medium. Future generations who have enjoyed a lifetime with television and modern conveniences such as automobiles, washing machines and dish washers may have no trouble using them as they grow old. Many of the social activities of older men and women are influenced by what was enjoyed in their youth rather than today.

Surprising facts are always coming to light. It is generally agreed that walking slows down with age, but the amount of time given to it does not. One study of groups of older people still working showed that they walked regularly more than the younger staff; again, the present generation of elderly people has been less accustomed to automobiles.

New findings of this sort do not cause embarrassment, but the idea that old people have sexual interests, and may even be sexually active, tends to be rejected automatically by younger people, particularly where their parents are concerned. Yet although sexual activity may decline with age, a new partner coming on the scene may change things dramatically. It is not only unkind but also unwise not to recognize the sexual needs of old people and to think of a blossoming of late romance as unhealthy. This is an area that we go into more fully in Chapter 3.

So, we may conclude that old people are infinitely varied, even if they share certain physical characteristics, such as greying hair and wrinkled skin. They become shorter and in a strange way approach the stage of intersex, an old man ceasing to shave regularly as his voice becomes piping, while an old lady's chin sprouts hair and her voice deepens. These are not important changes. As carers our concern must be with the preservation of personality and vigour, just as we seek to promote these attributes in a child. We hope the advice we give will help you achieve this aim. Rather than this book being an instruction manual, it should be considered a chart or ground plan for you to proceed confidently, learning for yourself the best way of caring for your own relative.

13

2 DECIDING ON HOME CARE

Your first concern when taking over responsibility for an elderly relative is how much and what type of care is needed. In this chapter we outline the options to help you decide which will be most suitable in your case.

Most of us have come across at least someone over eighty who is still capable of living alone. Despite being small and thin, many people of this age are wiry and surprisingly strong, with alert mental faculties. The only care they need is a regular visit by someone who can keep a watchful eye for anything unusual. Yet this is a responsibility to be taken seriously. Neglect of a lonely old person is often the cause of life-threatening illness.

The first signs that living alone is no longer possible for an elderly person may be minor – difficulty with day-to-day functions, for example, spilling hot drinks or taking longer to climb the stairs. There is a more urgent need for care when there has been:

- Bereavement, especially loss of a partner
- Loss as a result of illness, or removal, of a principal helper
- Sudden loss of capacity, such as a heart attack, stroke, major surgery, or mental failure
- Discharge from the hospital after a major operation.

These are situations when something has to be done immediately. But you can gain time to organize things by arranging temporary admission to a convalescent or nursing home. It is unusual in my experience for people to be prepared for these events, and when they happen the younger relatives need professional support. Among the factors you have to consider will be your own position. In the past it was unthinkable that anyone other than the family would care for an elderly parent. We must not assume that this was ideal. Usually there were few options, and especially in Western societies, old people were often treated with cruelty and neglect. Now we have a range of choices, from total care by the family to living in an institution such as a hospital, old people's home or hospice. Between these extremes are methods of shared care with medical personnel and assistants with some training, such as night sitters and volunteers.

14

Why should anyone care?

Only you can make the decision to play the major role in caring for someone else. Since it is so important and one that may affect the lives of others, it is not to be undertaken lightly.

It has been said that people no longer care for their elderly relatives in the wonderful way they did in the past. Younger people have become selfish and materialistic and cannot bother with their parents. It is not uncommon to hear old women speak bitterly about being neglected by their children, and it is only too easy to share their feelings – until, at least, you have heard the children's side of the story! Very often a different picture emerges, showing that the old complainer had never assumed the role of a true parent when it was required.

On both sides, then, the past relationship governs present feelings, and often children have an agonizing desire to help and support a loved parent at the end of his or her life. I knew two young women who regularly crossed the city in the rush hour to cook an evening meal for their mothers, even incurring some neglect of their husbands and children because of it. This is the simplest of motives, the return on an earlier investment of affection and emotion. There are of course a variety of others, ranging from a sense of cold duty, through being the only one available, to the less admirable motive of material reward.

Who is to care?

An unmarried only son or daughter will inevitably assume sole responsibility; this will be a daunting prospect, and in Chapter 7 we give advice on coping alone. Where more than one younger relative lives close, there is no formula as to who should do the caring. There is nothing laid down that says it must be the daughter rather than the son, or the youngest, or the eldest. Most adults have many commitments, so if several people can offer a home the burden may be shared to everyone's advantage. Preliminary discussions are all important to decide how much time and what particular skills each can contribute. Ideally, this will be harmoniously resolved into a roster for caring. But sometimes there is bitterness when one or other of those expected to care ducks out, or there is a possessiveness over the elder relative. I remember two Greek brothers fighting each other for the right to care exclusively for their old father! Where family tensions are difficult to resolve, a third party, trusted by all, such as a close friend or minister, can act as mediator.

The obvious mistake sometimes made is not to involve the old person concerned in all the important decisions. On one occasion, we had worked out a very careful and detailed plan of support for an old man and his chairbound wife, but when it was put to them the husband rejected it out of hand, and our effort was entirely wasted. We all have the right to be consulted about our future, both with near family and others such as doctors, social workers or lawyers. In this way anxieties on both sides, even about straightforward matters such as suitability of the accommodation, have an airing.

Making the move

The decision, sometimes a painful one, is how long you can continue visiting your relative at home, or whether a change is necessary now. Faced with her advancing frailty, you must decide how long will it be before a move must be made for her own safety and wellbeing. The house where she lives may be your childhood home too. It holds memories, like a time capsule, and you may regard its present state with pity or regret, or maybe you feel great affection for it and want those memories to be preserved. But whatever your feelings, the prime consideration must be its suitability as a home for your relative.

How does she manage to shop? What contact and help is provided by neighbours, and what social amenities does the neighbourhood provide? The chances are that if she is very old, friends and acquaintances will also be old, housebound or no longer alive.

Even more important, how does your relative look after the house and herself?

- Can she wash and bathe herself, and do her laundry?
- Is the toilet accessible? Can the flush be operated easily?
- How would help be summoned if she fell in the house – is there an alarm system or telephone?
- Can your relative keep the place clean, and are the electric outlets for connecting the vacuum cleaner easily reached?
- Is the place too big to heat so that your relative may skimp on food or clothing to pay the bills?
- If the home lacks the necessary conveniences but your relative wants to remain there, can improvements be made?

When moving has been accepted as a necessity in the forseeable future, but is not a matter of urgency, it is best to make the change gradually. Contact can increase steadily from an occasional, say monthly, visit or weekly telephone call, right up to constant day and night care. What starts as minimal involvement will intensify over time.

Good planning needs a realistic assessment of the possibilities, and experimentation. For instance, much can be gained by inviting your elderly relative to spend a limited time with you. We're all aware that you really don't know people until you live with them, and this may include your own mother after an interval of fifty years! Only by being under the same roof again can you learn how adaptable she is, and how your partner, children and other family members react. Remember, we are talking now about a home rather than an institution for the elderly,

16

about pride, possession, personality, sentiment and mutual respect. We are talking about territory.

How far can you see it through?

No one knows, of course, but the main factor will be your degree of motivation. The emotional bond between you and your relative provides the incentive through all the difficult times, so it must be sincere and strong. We have already said it will make the new arrangements much easier for everyone if you begin by looking realistically at how you are equipped. Previous experience is invaluable. Nursing comes naturally to some people who are practical, and have plenty of common sense. Most women with children have been put to the test of caring for sick children or a husband at some time. Many men have learned the job of running a household, looking after children and supporting their wife during pregnancy.

A most important requirement is good physical and mental health. Only the healthy can deal with irregular hours, physical effort and emotional strain, so if you are not confident about whether your health is good enough, it is wise to consult your family doctor. Consider too your mental qualities. Endurance will be needed, but it is also important to remain flexible even at difficult times, and to keep your sense of humour – for you may be sure you will often need it! Have you the love and patience necessary, and will it worry you if you are sometimes less than perfect?

Inevitably the act of caring involves giving up a lot in your present life. I have found in nine cases out of ten that people deeply engaged in caring do not seem to be aware of the sacrifices. Only later, perhaps, when the job is finished, are you able to sense the satisfaction it has brought you. Sacrificing other people, however, is a different business, so you must be sensitive to the needs of others who depend on you, and now allow them to feel neglected.

Making the right choice

To make this important decision as to how much long-term care you can give and whether you will need outside assistance you have to think about the following factors:

- The degree of dependency and behaviour of your relative
- Your own health
- The distance and time taken travelling to your relative's home
- Your doctor's estimate of your relative's present and future health
- The support of other family members
- Your understanding of the level of care needed
- Your financial resources

17

- The suitability of your home
- How you will tolerate restriction in your work, holidays, meeting friends
- The opportunities for relief care, breaks or holidays
- The likely duration of the commitment.

It is equally disastrous to undertake the task of caring on impulse and abandon it when confronted with the hard realities as it is to reject it out of hand because of its apparent enormity. This is the kind of choice which, if made unwisely, can have a destructive influence on the remainder of your adult life. So it is best taken with the help of someone experienced and concerned, but outside the immediate family. Such a person may be the family physician, a wise friend or minister, who will share the burden of decision making, and will have a different slant on the matter.

Minimizing resistance to change

Both your elderly relative and the other members of your family will find the new situation difficult. It is worth pausing for a moment to consider ways that resistance to change, and later failures, can be avoided. Here are some mistakes that are commonly made when there isn't sufficient planning:

- The purpose of change is not made clear; no one enjoys change for its own sake
- The people affected are not involved from the beginning
- There is poor communication, resulting in a misunderstanding or mistrust
- Habitual behaviour is ignored
- Resistance arises from a feeling of being pressured
- Anxiety is created over personal security; reassurance is needed
- Changing homes involves loss of your relative's self-esteem
- Conflict or competition is created between different members of the family.

A change in lifestyle involves learning new skills and altering attitudes. First, we have to decide how we should like things to be, then plan how we can make it happen. We must also make the plan clear from the beginning to the person to be cared for. Then we have to review the situation constantly to see everything is going according to plan.

How do you offer help?

A lot of tact and diplomacy are needed. Above all, old people must never be made to suspect interference, or that they are being taken over. You may be offended by a forthright refusal of your offer of a home, but equally you may be alarmed if your suggestions are taken up too readily by a relative willing to abandon a house and lifestyle all at once. Although the former situation is more likely, both will be avoided so long as you do not make an offer until all aspects have been weighed up realistically by you and your relative.

A proper concern, with such questions as, 'How do you do your washing?' or, 'What are you going to prepare for lunch today?' can bring about a shared understanding that there are deficiencies in your relative's lifestyle that can be rectified. Sometimes old people are thought to be obstinate, when in fact they are coping with overbearing rudeness such as someone coming in and saying, 'This place is filthy and needs tidying up', or, 'Why don't you eat something more nourishing?' If on a regular visit you find that things have suddenly been neglected, then you should realize that this is almost certainly the result of illness. At this stage it is as well for you to arrange for a thorough medical check-up (see page 28).

What care is needed?
Careful thought is needed to decide what and how much care should be supplied. Over provision leads to dependency and is a more common fault than under provision, and can lead to the old person becoming a human pet. But if you think back to the basic needs, for good food, warmth and clothing, love and prestige, good housing, and an occasional luxury, you should arrive at the right balance. Every relationship is different, but the assessment of another's needs demands sensitivity and imagination. These may be predominantly physical, such as coping with reduced mobility, or emotional, such as feeling there is still a family bond, or social, such as the need for conversation or continued attendance at a social group. They are more likely to combine several of these aspects.

There are various options for achieving the right amount of care besides bringing your relative into your own home:

1. Home conversion If your relative is still reasonably independent but can no longer occupy or reach the upper floor of the home, this may be converted and rented out as an extra source of income. Such an arrangement provides some supervision, and a sense of security. Sometimes people's entire capital is locked up in their property, so their income remains insufficient for heating and feeding. You might make inquiries about what supplementary benefits are available in your area which would enable your relative to remain independent (see Chapter 9).

2. Specially-built homes In recent years there has been a marked improvement in residential and supervised homes for elderly people,

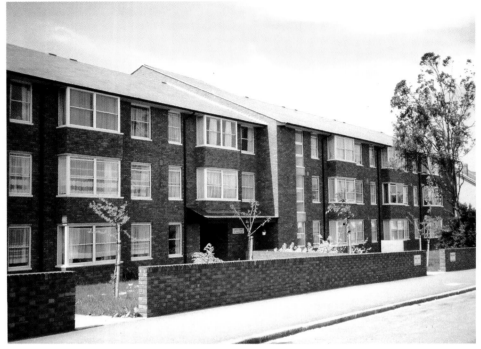

Purpose-built apartments allow privacy and independence – while communal facilities and a resident warden mean help is always available.

and these can be the ideal compromise between independence and total dependence. The idea is often advanced, almost as a dogma, that old people are happiest when left in their own homes, and that to move them is a recipe for disaster. This was probably largely true in the days before there were the attractive alternatives of specially-built homes. With their obvious convenience and a new generation of old people more used to travel and social mobility, moving is often a great success. Of course, old people do not initially want to be removed from their familiar surroundings. Usually there is a feeling of better the devil you know than the one you don't. I have now had experience of many transfers to specially-built accommodation, and this has shown me that most old people welcome it, but only after we have discussed every aspect sympathetically and at length, and they have had the opportunity first of inspecting their new home. It was surely the failure to take time on this in the past that often gave rise to the belief in the obstinacy of old people.

3. Old people's homes and hospitals These are probably the least desirable of the choices. One of the reasons for deciding against a long-stay hospital or a home for the elderly is the loss of the lifegiving qualities of independence, and the effects on the personality, called 'institutionalization'. We have all seen, if not at first hand, pictures of old people who have lost any sense of purpose, just sitting around staring into space. They become entirely passive and all former features of their personalities are lost.

Of course, this is not universal and many hospitals and homes succeed in keeping old people active, mobile and involved, even though this is more difficult than in a family home. The reverse is true too, and something to be carefully guarded against. Old people can quite easily become institutionalized in their own home, or in yours, if they do not feel they belong or contribute any more.

Having an elderly relative in your own home is not the only or necessarily the best answer. But it is still the most common solution and often the most successful. I concentrate on the practical aspects of this arrangement later because, as I have said before, a comfortable physical environment goes a very long way towards harmony for the whole family. First I shall talk about adapting the home itself to make it the right environment for your relative as well as for you and your family.

Whose home is it to be?
You will have to decide whether your relative comes to live in your house or whether you move into his or hers. The former is more likely, although sometimes the relative's home is larger and a move by the younger generation is not too disrupting to family life and jobs. Then this is a good solution.

Whichever you choose, it is important to consider above all its suitability for your relative. And if it was his or hers, the adaptations you make will have to be done with tact and consideration. In recent times a generation gap has developed, with younger people living in different circumstances from their elders, and it is easy for them to criticize old people's surroundings as dingy and unsuitable. Yet older people find the bright wall hangings and loud music enjoyed by the young intolerable. As with all aspects of the new arrangement, you will probably have to compromise over decorations.

How suitable is the home?
Your aged parent may still occupy a rambling family home in its own grounds, while you live in a modern apartment. Even so, the alternative of moving into your relative's home may not be suitable. While the old family home is spacious enough, it may lack modern conveniences, or have become neglected; the neighbourhood may have become run down. In this case the property, or both properties, might be sold to provide another, more convenient house. A popular trend is to add an extension to an existing home.

21

More often it is necessary or possible only to make minor changes to the house to suit your relative's needs. In the UK you can ask for a visit from a specialized adviser from your local municipal government, who will give expert advice not only in matters such as safety and insulation, but also information on improvement grants that can be made for older homes. In North America and Australia, cash assistance is available rather than a service (see Chapter 9).

Modifications that might be needed
You should think about the following areas carefully and decide what modifications should be made to allow maximum mobility and safety.

Heating
- Safety of appliances, for example, heat guards, flues, electrical installations, switches, wires
- Economy, reduction of heat loss, insulation
- The need for extra heating to achieve a minimum safe temperature for anyone in advanced old age with poor mobility and illness, of 65°F (18.3°C). In the UK insulation and heating grants are available for home owners.

Lighting
- **Illumination** Make sure there is good lighting where it is most needed, for example, on staircases, over sinks, in cellars and porches, and outside where there are steps and at garbage disposal areas.

  Remember, well-directed, close lighting is best. It is more efficient to have a 60 watt lamp at your elbow for close work than a 200 watt bulb four yards away in the ceiling.

- **Installation** Old premises may need rewiring, or there may be a fire hazard. Consult an approved electrician. Where plugs are inserted and removed frequently, for example, in the kitchen, it is helpful to position them at waist height.

Ventilation
Old people often take up their quarters in a small room and barricade the doors and windows against heat loss. Oxygen is prevented from entering and carbon dioxide levels rise, producing drowsiness. Whereas the old-fashioned fireplace, which is still sometimes used, assisted ventilation by drawing air into the room, a gas or solid fuel appliance needs an outlet to stop carbon monoxide building up in the atmosphere.

Fire hazards

Old people sometimes become less aware of their surroundings through impaired vision and loss of sense of smell. They need to be reminded of fire hazards and to take precautions:

- Always use a lighter rather than matches
- Warn against smoking in bed, and while dozing in a chair
- Buy a fire extinguisher and inform neighbours where it is installed
- Do not store inflammables such as turpentine indoors
- Buy flame-resistant night clothes and chair covers
- Never carry heaters from room to room. Install them against a wall, away from cross draughts. Be very careful when filling a heater, and have it serviced regularly.

Accessibility

Old people are liable to feel giddy when they bend down or straighten up, and when they stretch or have to climb on a ladder or chair. Place kitchen cupboards at a level where everything is within easy reach. Keep all cupboards and closets uncluttered and free of unnecessary items which prevent easy access.

Floors

The ideal floor surface is even and non-slip. Replace old floor coverings that have curled or split. Keep the floor clear of other hazards, such as misplaced door stops or dropped balls of wool. Do not allow too much furniture to clutter rooms, and discourage your relative from using it as a support, since it may be unsteady. It is better to keep central areas clear and use a lightweight tripod walking aid.

The bedroom

The position of this room is all-important. Your relative's bedroom may at present be upstairs. For anyone with a debilitating condition, such as heart disease, climbing stairs is an aggravating factor. Although moving the bedroom downstairs is the best solution, habits are hard to change. A trial period of sleeping downstairs usually persuades even the most reluctant old person of the benefits.

The height of the bed is important. Old people find it easier to get in and out of a high bed rather than a low one. Another item to consider carefully is the mattress. One that is too soft also makes getting out of bed very difficult. Many old people like to sleep in cold bedrooms, and if this is true of your relative you should see that there is sufficient warmth in the bed. An electric overblanket, provided it is absolutely safe, is an excellent means of maintaining even body warmth.

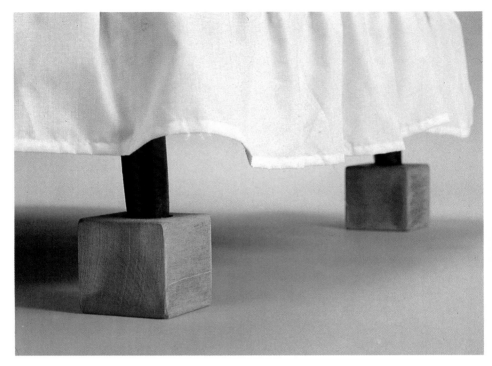
If your relative finds bending difficult, raise the bed on wooden blocks.

The toilet must of course be considered in relation to the bedroom, and a good general rule is that it should not be more than fifteen paces away from the bed. This may mean installing a new toilet, although a portable commode would be a cheaper alternative.

Getting up at night can be a hazard, so you should arrange for a night light, which consumes a minimum of electricity, to be kept in your relative's bedroom.

The bathroom
The dangers to guard against in the bathroom are falling, slipping, scalding and electrocution:

1. Have a handrail placed vertically beside the bath.

2. Most modern baths have non-slip surfaces; if yours does not, buy a special mat held down by suction pads. These are available from hardware stores.

3. If your relative has frail or arthritic limbs and cannot sit right in or get out of the bath by kneeling, you will have to provide a bath seat. There are hoists that lift handicapped people up and into the

bath but these can only be used if there is someone available to operate them. These hoists are also of course very expensive.

4. Warn your relative never to get into a bath without first testing the temperature.

5. On no account have an electric heater in the bathroom, unless it is fixed high on the wall, out of reach.

The toilet

Having satisfactory toilet arrangements is central to your relative's comfort. Here are some important points to consider when making the toilet as easy to use as possible:

- Is the approach well lit, safe and obstacle-free?

- Does your relative need to use stairs to get to it, and if so would a handrail be useful?

- Is there a heat source so that cold does not act as a deterrent and lead to irregular bowel movements?

A removable seat is the simplest way to convert the bath if your relative cannot sit right in; a firmly fixed handrail is vital for anyone likely to slip.

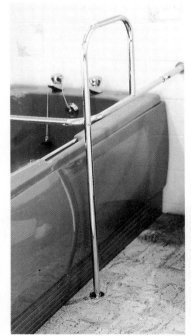
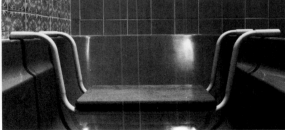

- Is it easy to enter in a hurry, and is the door wide enough to allow entry when using a walking aid?
- If your relative lives in an apartment, is the toilet shared, and with how many?
- If he or she has moved home recently, does he know the way to the toilet, and where light switches and handles are?
- Would a sign on the door be helpful?
- If the toilet is small, would it help to rehang the door so that it opens outwards rather than inwards?
- Does the door open and close easily?
- If the old person is arthritic, can he or she manage the light switch, or would a cord pull be helpful?
- Can he reach to raise and lower the seat?
- Is the seat at the right height so that he can sit and rise easily?
- Are handrails needed for extra support? Remember that muscle tone is reduced after sleep, impairing the ability to raise the body weight.
- Can your relative operate the flushing system and the door handle?
- Should there be an alarm or call system to give confidence?
- Is the floor covering easy to clean?

The lists of points to check and the adaptations that may need making seem endless. Many are simply done, and if you are able to make at least the majority of these changes, you will have a home that is eminently suited to your relative, and comfortable for you too. In the next chapter I explain how making the best of minor disabilities will maintain your relative's mobility and independence, and so enhance his or her enjoyment of life.

3 DELAYING THE INEVITABLE

The main reasons an older person may no longer be able to live alone are reduced mobility and the risks of illness, which with increasing age are difficult to fight off. In this chapter I explain which are the usual disabilities and illnesses and what symptoms to look out for, and I suggest ways that good health and independence can be preserved as long as possible.

These days illness and disability in later life result far more often from lifestyle than from those old diseases such as tuberculosis and polio. While there is in all of us a certain programme of aging, with events like puberty and the menopause occurring sooner or later, an unhealthy way of life will accelerate the start of the aging diseases. For instance, everyone knows that smoking is associated with certain heart diseases of a degenerative kind. If you live long enough, such degeneration is to be expected, but by advancing the start of these diseases to middle life, the likelihood of fatal or disabling consequences is much higher.

Attention to health needs
It is never too late to start on a healthy lifestyle. Although damage may have been done by harmful activities, better health and a sense of wellbeing will result from giving up bad habits, misuse of drugs and alcohol, and smoking. As principal carer for an older relative you are probably in the best position to suggest these changes, and tactful yet firm intervention in late middle age may even prevent serious disease in later life. The fact that you care should be an incentive for your relative to respond. Old people who don't have anyone to care for them often see no reason to alter their ways: if there is no one else to consider, who can blame them for selfishness?

Dangers of neglect
Self-neglect is not uncommon in the elderly, and it very often arises from loneliness and depression. Of course, there are those who have always isolated themselves, and who survive in rather squalid conditions, which they are used to and find perfectly acceptable. We are concerned here with people to whom self-neglect is recent and out of character. This is a symptom of illness rather than a way of life. The danger is that it is ever-increasing, becoming a downward spiral that ends in hopelessness and despair. Everything becomes too much effort,

27

so that water is left running, and lights burning. The senses of taste and smell become less acute with age; sensitivity to cold and heat are blunted. Some of the signs of self-neglect to look out for are:

- An odour of urine
- Untidiness
- An attitude of neglect, acceptance, hopelessness and lack of motivation
- Soiled linen accumulating
- Changing clothes infrequently or wearing night clothes all the time
- Not taking prescribed medicine or hoarding drugs such as sedatives, tranquillizers or sleeping pills.

No wonder depressed old people are thought to have become demented, when in fact all they need is often simply love and affection, and help with the daily chores. Caring means constantly checking the way your relative is living, knowing there will be a gradual decline, and making sure that medical checks are made and proper medical care is given as it is needed. When there are clues that your relative is unwell, suffering from the problems I have listed above, you should talk to the family doctor. As long as minor ailments are kept in control, your relative's independence can be preserved.

The check-up
I believe this is a useful measure, especially for older people. Its purpose is to detect early signs of disease in the hope that it can be slowed down, or even reversed. The main functions such as heart, blood pressure, eyesight and hearing are checked. An elevated blood pressure may be discovered, for instance, at a time when one feels perfectly fit. If this is controlled it can delay the onset of blood vessel diseases.

Some people argue that check-ups do as much harm as they do good, and that the medical treatment can even reduce the quality of life. Some doctors are too eager to prescribe regular treatment that may not be entirely necessary. When all the arguments for and against are weighed up, I think the check-up is money well spent if it will lead to modifications in lifestyle. And this applies perhaps better to the old than the young. In my experience older people care desperately about the quality of the time remaining, while the young feel they are able to play Russian roulette with health hazards and find it more difficult to change.

For people over seventy-five, I would recommend an annual check.

How do you define disability?
From the age of sixty onwards, there is a sharp rise in the chances of

your having some disability. Over the age of eighty-five, two-thirds of the population are disabled in one way or another. That is, they are unable to do what they want, or what they need to do. Always remember that disability is related to a necessary function such as sight, hearing or mobility rather than a particular illness. The same condition will affect people differently according to their way of life. For instance, a musician but not an artist would be disabled by deafness, while a shaking hand that might just be a nuisance to some people would prevent an artist from painting. Someone already using a wheelchair could surmount a leg amputation with little change of lifestyle.

The progress and severity of a disease also determines whether it will involve disability. Some diseases such as an acute chest infection can be cured, and the progress of certain cancers is so slow in old people that it is not always the cause of death. Certain forms of heart and vessel disease, or mental illness, develop slowly and surely, and at present there is no effective treatment.

Multiple disability

An old person's disability is hardly ever due to one disease only. For example, it is not sufficient simply to blame 'arthritis' or 'rheumatism' when your relative finds walking painful. As with all physical or mental failings it is essential to arrange a thorough check-up by a doctor who is experienced in geriatric medicine. This may show that one disorder masks another. Say someone's mobility has been restricted by Parkinson's disease, but, because this can now be successfully treated, he becomes quite mobile again. Now he complains of a pain in the chest and shortness of breath, yet while he was sitting all the time these symptoms of heart disease did not bother him. Finding out the whole truth is vitally important.

Coping with disability

Disablement may finally drive old people to give up living on their own, or to seek help from others, so it must be resisted. Many disabilities can be prevented or at least delayed by early diagnosis and treatment, or by abandoning unhealthy habits. But when a certain degree of disability has to be accepted, the remaining ability can always be built on. An old person's fighting spirit is perhaps the most important asset and in my view has some of the quality seen in a wild animal. You should be careful not to domesticate your relative by taking away independence and preventing him or her from doing things. Old people are often highly inventive in overcoming disabilities, and though their efforts may seem strange or poorly worked out, it is best to leave them to continue as long as possible. I say this because of my conviction that every time you encourage a disabled person to do something within his or her capability, you help recovery and lessen disability.

What should your attitude be? With people you love, you often have a feeling of tenderness and pity when confronted with their old age and disability. In themselves, these sentiments are not enough. You need to match the fighting spirit and motivation of an older person. Indeed, true understanding requires a tough attitude on the part of the principal helper. A strong supportive framework with clear objectives must be planned.

If goals are not set, or they are unrealistic, all that can be expected in the end is bitterness, frustration and depression. The following are essential for maintaining health and fitness:

- Keeping to the diet advised by the doctor or dietitian (see page 46)

- Doing any exercise that has been recommended by the doctor; this will probably be a gentle, regular programme such as a short daily walk or some circulation or mobility exercises suitable for the less able (see the photographs on page 52)

- Following faithfully whatever medical treatments may have been prescribed; most elderly people have to take some pills, either for high blood pressure or arthritis, or maybe for a heart condition. These can be effective only if they are taken in the right doses at the right times.

Above all, you should tackle any disabilities with energy and optimism. Even though people with a permanent disability have to accept their situation, and for them we naturally feel sympathy, we must not allow matters to rest there. There is no place for defeatism, for there is always something more that can be done. A 5 per cent improvement in walking distance, or breathing capacity, a little more sleep, a reduction of pain – these add up to an encouraging feeling of achievement all round.

Later in this book we shall be considering the four giants which threaten old people, all of them beginning with the letter I:

Instability

Immobility

Incontinence

Intellectual failure.

They require special consideration; but let us first look at the common complaints. These are often overlooked, and yet they too can have a cumulative serious effect on your relative's health.

30

Common health problems

In old people, ill health usually announces itself stealthily. As in childhood, a disease may first be noticed by an alteration in behaviour. Even doctors and nurses sometimes respond to some minor complaints, such as someone feeling 'off colour', by saying, 'Well, what can you expect at your age?' People often resign themselves to the idea that aches and pains are an expected part of growing old, and may even be glad to have an excuse not to admit to fear of a disease. So let us examine some of the common problems that may affect your relative's health and see how they might best be understood and treated.

Many of the same symptoms are caused by different conditions, so when you are trying to find the root of the problem you must spend some time investigating and not jump to conclusions too soon. Whenever in doubt about your relative's health you should consult your doctor.

When an elderly relative first moves into a new home some mental distress at the upheaval and worry about how the future is going to work out is inevitable. It is not uncommon for this anxiety to progress to a condition that needs medical attention – and the symptoms of this type of anxiety are easily noticeable.

Anxiety and depression

We often imagine that old age is a time of peace and contentment. In fact, when mental and physical powers are declining, old people feel anxious because they are losing control. In more naturalistic and agricultural communities, where social patterns remain familiar, old people suffer less from this anxiety. But with the changed behaviour in present Western society old people may feel isolated, even in the heart of a loving family. Outside the family, the pace of life has speeded up to such an extent that they feel totally alienated. I am not speaking here of people who have always been worriers. They will never change. The ones to be concerned about are those who become anxious for the first time in middle life or old age. This sort of anxiety often leads to depression, which though it has similar symptoms, is a separate condition and more deep-rooted.

The symptoms most noticeable in old people are:

- Insomnia and continual tiredness
- Loss of appetite and weight loss, or alternatively compulsive eating
- Feelings of guilt
- Difficulty in decision making
- Feeling sad.

31

In a true state of depression, the symptoms are more intense and require medical attention.

How do you alleviate anxiety and depression?
Unfortunately, the closer you are to someone, the more difficult it is to be able to help. You often hear people saying, 'Come on! Snap out of it! Pull yourself together!' and so on. What is really being said is, 'I don't like you the way you are. So behave as I do. You are spoiling things.' Of course this is quite cruel, and only designed to make the condition worse, and the sufferer feel more guilty.

A real desire to understand, an arm around the shoulder, a sharing of dark fears, perhaps of loneliness, death and hopelessness, and even shedding tears together, may bring respite. But this will probably be only temporary, for true depression is an illness. It is one that responds well to medical treatment if not allowed to continue too long. If treatment is delayed, the symptoms already mentioned – loss of appetite, altered behaviour and sleep – take their toll physically and mentally. Ask your doctor's advice early rather than late.

Insomnia
Sleep becomes a problem with old people for a variety of reasons. Whereas a young person takes about ten minutes to go off to sleep, by the age of seventy it takes about twenty-five minutes. Frequent waking is common, and because the stage of very deepest sleep is significantly reduced in old people they may feel dissatisfied not only with the quantity, but also with the quality of their sleep. Yet often elderly people are getting enough sleep, only in a different way from when they were young. The pattern changes as we grow older and long periods of sleep are replaced by more frequent, shorter naps, many of them during the day. As a result the total sleep period may not change greatly. Nevertheless, worry about insomnia prompts a huge number of old people to take sleeping pills. A recent study showed that 15 per cent of men and 30 per cent of women regularly take sleeping pills, and it has been estimated that 30 per cent of all these are consumed by the elderly population. This is liable to lead to an unnecessary dependence on these drugs. As yet, no pill has been developed that will restore normal sleep, so taking pills should not be encouraged.

Some old people want to kick the sleeping pill habit, which often originates from a stay in hospital. The best way to do this is by a gradual reduction in dosage and prolonging the interval between doses, while paying attention to comfort and security and rewarding achievement with praise.

What causes lack of sleep?   If your relative is constantly having trouble sleeping, consider these as the possible reasons:

- There are many pains and discomforts of the elderly which may not worry young people, such as a full bladder, distended rectum, cramps, skin irritations, coughs, palpitations and heart pain

- Anxiety and depression are common in old age

- Simple causes are often overlooked such as the stimulating effect of tea or coffee drunk late at night, or even trying to work out the solution to a crossword puzzle

- Although naps are normal, your relative should not be constantly dropping off to sleep at odd times. This may be a sign of diabetes or failing kidney function and should be checked out.

Old people are like children in needing routine sleeping times and preparation for them. Always ensure that conditions are favourable by checking the temperature of the room, the humidity, noise level and lighting.

Anxieties should be talked about. Very often an older person is concerned with simple and immediate things such as fear of waking others when using the toilet at night, but if the anxiety is more deep-rooted, for example, a concern with being a burden to others, simple reassurance will not be sufficient. Watch out for a state of anxiety or depression (see above). Very early waking is the characteristic sleep disturbance of depressed people. They will lie in bed and ruminate over their failures and unworthiness, and you will find yourself unable to dislodge these feelings of self-reproach. Then you should speak to the family doctor or geriatrician.

Here is a useful list I distribute to people who are having sleep problems.

1. Before going to bed make sure you are pleasantly tired.

2. You won't sleep if you are in pain, hungry (a milky drink can help), or too full with a heavy meal, or if you have been dozing or physically inactive during the day.

3. Gentle exercise (like a short walk) will help you to relax and to feel genuinely tired – but don't overdo it – and do make it regular (it needn't be taken just before you go to bed).

4. Try to establish a simple routine every night on going to bed – habit helps you to sleep.

5. A warm drink, a warm bath and a good book (not too exciting) can work wonders.

6. Try to avoid alcohol, especially early in the evening. You may drop off by the fire or in front of the television and wake up restless halfway through the night.

7. Once in bed, make sure you are comfortable – not too hot or too cold, with a firm (not hard) mattress.
8. Fresh (not freezing) air, and as little noise as possible, will also help.
9. If you haven't been sleeping well for a long time (weeks) or if you feel tired every morning, in spite of this advice, talk things over with your doctor.
10. Above all, don't worry about the amount of sleep you are going to get – you can manage on surprisingly little.

Very often, old people who have been poor sleepers settle down well when they stay with caring relatives. Like children, they respond to a sense of security, and sleeping drugs may be given up.

Fatigue
Feeling tired is often the reason given by old people for not being more physically or mentally active. The causes may be psychological or physical:

- A reflection of boredom and depression in those recently retired, especially if retirement was compulsory, or after a bereavement
- An anxiety leading to loss of sleep
- The poor quality of the diet or too much alcohol
- The effect of prescribed or other drugs, such as a 'cold remedy'
- A wide range of diseases such as diabetes, anaemia, thyroid failure, chronic infection, cancer or heart disease.

Listlessness may lead to not eating enough, apathy, neglect and a chair-bound state of dependency. Make sure the true causes are discovered so that the correct treatment is given.

Headache
Headaches tend to be dismissed as trivial, especially as some people are prone to them all their lives. Persistent headaches that start in later life are an indication of illness:

- Your relative may have had a recent head injury or eye trouble; ask particularly whether there is a blurring of vision, or if the headache comes on regularly after reading
- The blood vessels in the temple region may feel tender; this is caused by inflammation of the arteries and you should consult your doctor immediately

- Pain in the nerves of the face and neck are caused by neuralgia and this produces headaches
- Very occasionally the bones of the skull have enlarged, causing a condition called Paget's disease
- In poorly ventilated rooms heating appliances may release the poisonous gas, carbon monoxide, and increased concentrations can produce unpleasant headaches in the region of the forehead
- Insufficient sleep, anxiety and depression give old people headaches, just as they do the young.

So, headaches can be the symptoms of a number of serious conditions. Diagnosis is important and a timely visit to the doctor is essential.

Poor appetite

I am often asked to prescribe a tonic to restore an old person's appetite. Even if there were such a medicine, before I agreed to give it I should always want to know the reason for appetite loss. Although not everyone eats less when older, generally this is so and is nothing to worry about. But you will not fail to notice if there has been a sudden change in choice and quantity of the food taken. The reason may simply be poorly fitting dentures: while not reducing the intake they will limit choice and lead to foods such as fresh vegetables and fruits being avoided. These are important sources of vitamins and fibre, so if this is the cause, see that your relative's dentures are adjusted.

Depression, for reasons already mentioned, such as enforced retirement, bereavement, emotional disturbance through family disagreement, a feeling of being unwanted – will destroy appetite.

Another cause is excessive alcohol and tobacco consumption. If this is the case, you will see signs of self-neglect.

Maybe none of the above applies. Then you should look for physical reasons, such as difficulty in swallowing, altered bowel habit, internal pains, abdominal distension. These are all accompanied by weight loss, and often lethargy. They may be caused by a number of gastrointestinal troubles or other illness, and you should consult your doctor about them.

Does loss of appetite matter? This is not usually a symptom of a serious condition. If you have established that your relative is healthy, you should within reason allow him or her to eat food that is appealing. Because they are no longer developing physically older people need far less food than the young and they will get sufficient nourishment from as little as 1500 calories per day, provided this is in a varied diet of fresh foods.

You needn't and shouldn't always check or change what your relative is eating but you should at least guard against an unrelieved diet of, say, white bread, margarine and a sweet spread washed down with a sugary drink. Old people usually like well-flavoured foods, so it is a good idea sometimes to tempt a flagging appetite with spicy or ethnic foods presented attractively – of course keeping sugar, salt and saturated fats to the minimum (see also page 46 for advice on what to eat).

Constipation

This often becomes a problem for old people. Let me first point out that constipation has nothing to do with frequency of bowel movements but with the difficulty of passing a hard, dry movement. As far as frequency is concerned, anything between three times daily to once every three days is considered normal; although many older people were trained to have a daily movement and think it is necessary to maintain this by taking a laxative – a habit which I would discourage (see below).

There are a number of reasons for constipation: especially reduced intake of roughage (fibre in fruit and vegetables), insufficient fluid intake, weakening of the muscles and lack of exercise. If allowed to continue, constipation can become a serious condition. It can cause mental confusion, particularly at night, and it may mean your relative has to be admitted to the hospital. Problems to do with the bowels are always a source of embarrassment to elderly people, and your relative will probably be reluctant to tell you about being constipated. So if you suspect trouble, try to find out as tactfully as you can.

Any changes in normal bowel habits or the passing of blood or mucus should be reported to your doctor. Hard stools can sometimes have a ball valve action and produce involuntary opening of the bowel, so that loose movements flow around it, giving the impression of diarrhoea. Breaking up and removing the mass may require the skills of a home nurse.

Laxatives I do not recommend using laxatives to relieve constipation. It is better to increase roughage in the diet and drink enough fluid every day (see page 49). Laxatives create dependency and can have unpleasant and painful effects. If absolutely necessary, buy the fibre-based type rather than a severe drug. Your pharmacist will be able to guide you.

In any case, it is important to try and prevent excessive concern about bowel action. It can be obsessional, or even become delusional; alternatively, it may be associated with depression.

Breathing problems

It is to be expected that your relative will become short of breath after exercising, climbing stairs, carrying heavy packages. This is not dangerous provided the normal pulse rate (70-80 beats per minute) is restored after two to three minutes' rest; indeed it is heart-strengthening to keep up a certain amount of exercise (see page 50). However, you should constantly be aware of the possibility of disease. The important signs are:

- Unnatural tiredness
- Shortage of breath
- A persistent cough, especially at night
- Pain in the chest
- A blue colour of the face, especially around the lips.

The reasons for persistent breathlessness are usually diseases of the lungs and airways, and heart disease. Many smokers have a long history of bronchitis, so that the duration of symptoms is an important consideration in finding the cause. Bronchial asthma is another condition that is likely to have started earlier in life.

Other factors play a part too. For instance, as we age our chest wall becomes more rigid, reducing the chest expansion that allows deep breathing. Old people with a bent back are even more restricted in their breathing. Being overweight places a burden on heart and lungs, and anaemia reduces the distribution of oxygen to the body tissues. Finally the emotions, being closely linked with the rate and depth of breathing, can be a cause of breathlessness.

Whatever the cause, there are ways of improving matters. A reduction in weight will help people with bronchitis, emphysema and heart disease. Further improvement may be achieved by physiotherapy aimed at teaching abdominal breathing, how to cough, postural drainage and good posture.

Smokers should be encouraged to give up. There are those who think it unkind to advise old people to stop smoking. Of course, they must have a choice, and they must weigh up the pleasure of smoking against the restriction of activity. But they cannot take an informed decision without being aware of all the dangers. The breathlessness is due largely to partial asphyxia caused by carbon monoxide in the inhaled smoke displacing much of the oxygen carried by the red blood cells. The added risks of heart disease and lung cancer may already be known, but should be pointed out to heavy smokers.

Dizziness and falling

As many as 50 per cent of people over seventy suffer from dizziness. This is often puzzling, and for elderly people it's a frightening experience, and enough to undermine self-confidence. There are innumerable causes, the most common being:

1. Disturbances of the balance organ in the inner ear, and its various connections in the nervous system
2. Restriction of bloodflow through the brain (including circulatory problems); this may be due to interference with arteries running into the brain along the neck. Turning the head may reduce blood-flow to the back part of the brain
3. Sudden alteration of the heartbeat rhythm also reduces the blood-flow to the brain
4. Disturbances of vision
5. Alterations of blood pressure.

In fact, because there are so many possible causes you must consult your doctor if your relative suffers from attacks of dizziness. Special diagnostic tests will probably be necessary and your observations are likely to be extremely valuable. For instance, dizziness and falling is one of the early signs of Parkinson's disease, and you may have noticed at the same time changes in speed of movement and speech, which would support this diagnosis. Or there may have been a head injury which your relative has forgotten about, or a recent tendency to take more alcohol, which he or she wishes to conceal.

At all events, falling must be regarded as a symptom of an illness. It is not sufficient to pick your relative up and decide that he is all right because he hasn't injured himself.

Failing sight
All warning signs of failing sight should be heeded. Too often poor eyesight has come about through neglecting regular eye examinations, so important after the age of fifty. Elderly people often persist in seeking new glasses when they really need a good assessment by an eye specialist. Most eye conditions cannot be cured, but early diagnosis will allow for effective control.

Among the common conditions in the elderly are cataract and macular degeneration. Both of these are the result of aging. Cataract is a clouding of the eye lens so that vision becomes hazy, and bright lights dazzle. For many elderly people the deterioration is not so bad that medical treatment is necessary. Only when day-to-day functioning becomes impossible will an eye specialist recommend an operation to remove the lens. Make sure your relative has good strong lighting for reading, but avoids dazzling light by wearing tinted glasses in strong sunlight, and the cataract should not be too troublesome.

If an operation is recommended, it may involve anything from forty-

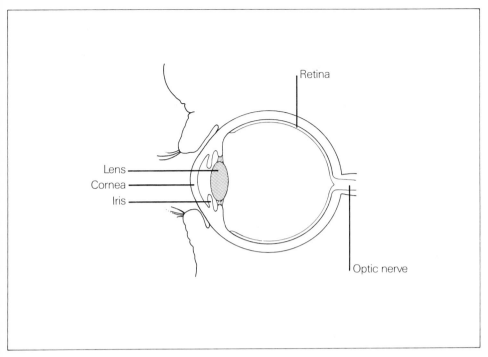

With a cataract the lens becomes opaque, making vision hazy.

eight hours to two weeks in the hospital, depending on the type. The lens will be replaced by an implanted lens, glasses or a contact lens, whichever is most suitable for your relative (contact lenses are often too difficult for old people to manage). The operation is nearly always successful and results in greatly improved sight. It is nothing to fear.

Macular degeneration is caused by the dying away of cells at the back of the retina, where images are received, so that central vision is affected and eventually may be lost. Around one in four people over sixty-five have a degree of macular degeneration. This is more difficult to adjust to than cataract, and unfortunately there is no cure for it. The one comfort is that this is only partial loss of vision, and by using peripheral vision your relative will still see to walk and be able to read by moving the head.

Glaucoma is another common eye problem of the elderly. Its detection is essential, and those whose near relatives have had the condition are especially likely to develop it. This is a state of raised pressure within the eyeball, which can be easily treated, usually by eyedrops, sometimes by operation. It is vital that medical treatment is followed to avoid later blindness.

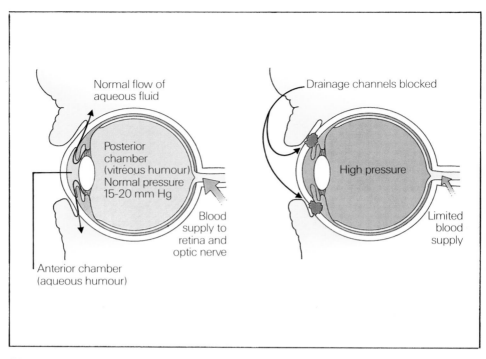

With glaucoma, pressure builds up in the eye because of the drainage being blocked.

If your relative has diabetes, you will already know that the eyesight is at risk, and careful control of the condition is essential to preserve it.

Should your relative unfortunately lose his or her sight, registration with your national blind or partially sighted organization is advisable. Blind people receive instruction on dressing, washing and cooking. They can apply for special aids such as a guide dog service, the talking book services, cassettes and telephone installation. For the partially sighted, visual aids such as hand magnifiers, telescopes and large print books are invaluable.

Further useful information on eye problems can be found in *Eyes: Their problems and treatments* by Michael Glasspool, FRCS, also in this series.

Deafness

Over the age of sixty your ability to detect high frequency sound is reduced. This particularly affects hearing consonants like t and s, so that speech begins to sound indistinct. I would advise you strongly to watch out for the beginnings of hearing loss in your friends and relatives. This can easily be done by speaking in different parts of the room, at different sound levels, without any appearance of formal testing.

You should never shout at old people. The increased volume of sound does nothing to alter the distortion. Thus the hearing aids that work as amplifiers, although useful for some forms of deafness, do not help this common type of old age deafness. What you are saying may be mixed in with extraneous noises going on at the same time. Whereas the old type of aid, called an ear trumpet, could be rotated towards the source of the sound, this is not the case with modern aids. Perhaps that is why so many of them are put away in drawers and not used! Old people are often persuaded to part with large amounts of money by smart salesmen who promise restored hearing.

While we seem to be drawn sympathetically to help the blind, the deaf receive much less patience and understanding. People who are becoming deaf are often aware of this sense of hostility and react by becoming suspicious and ill-tempered. They may in the end become frankly paranoid. I have even seen elderly couples fall out for the first time after their golden wedding because one of them has developed deafness which the other believes to have been acquired as a sort of convenient escape.

Hearing is very largely a cerebral function. Old people are unable to follow either rapid speech or complex forms of expression because of slowing up of the ability to interpret what they hear. They lose out in social gatherings as they cannot easily follow one conversation taking

Reading aids: a high-powered magnifying glass on a stand and, *below*, a plastic magnifying sheet is very effective held 4 in (10 cm) from the page.

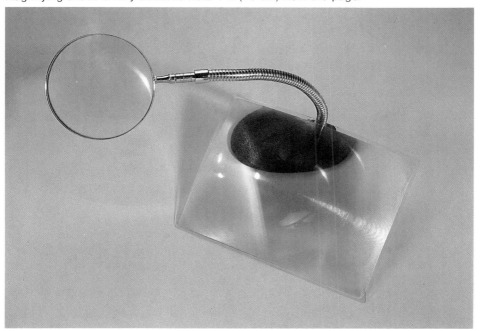

place among many. Communication with them should be slow and simple, something we recognize naturally with children.

You should also indicate in other ways what you are trying to say, by squeezing a hand, offering a caressing hand, or touching. So, if you want to communicate effectively with a deaf person, it is best to sit down or kneel by the chair, so that your face is in the light and at the same level as the listener's. Wait until he or she is alert and ready, and then speak slowly and clearly, accentuating the consonants. Not only will your expression and gestures convey much of your meaning, but you will be able to detect in the eyes of the listener how well you have been understood.

Finally, you can always write down difficult meanings, when all else has failed. Sometimes you may need to ask your relative to modulate his or her voice: old people often raise their voice when they cannot hear well themselves. This can be very embarrassing at times!

Backache
There are so many causes for this most common of complaints that careful investigation is extremely important:

1. First, there are all the causes that afflict younger people, such as muscle strain or slipped disc
2. All old people suffer from thinning of the bones, known as osteoporosis; this is due to a loss of calcium from middle life onwards and can be especially severe in women after the menopause. By the time people have reached their seventies the weakness of the bones may cause a weak and painful back. An increase in calcium intake, especially after the menopause, and in some cases replacement of the hormone oestrogen, are thought to delay osteoporosis, although it is never entirely avoided
3. Sometimes pain from abdominal organs extends to other places so that kidney pain and pain from the main blood vessels, and even the pancreas, may be felt in the back
4. There may be rheumatism or arthritis in the bones
5. Or deposits of cancer, usually from the breast in women, or the lung or prostate in men.

With so many possible causes, anyone with backache over the age of sixty needs radiographic examination for the diagnosis to be made. It is very unwise for any manipulative procedure (osteopathy or chirpractic) to be carried out before this has been done.

Foot problems
Elderly people will almost certainly develop foot problems – after all,

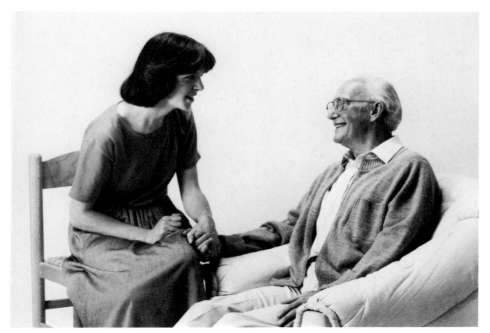
To make yourself understood, speak slowly and distinctly where your relative can see your face clearly.

the feet are subjected to heavy wear and tear throughout life, and being at the farthest extreme from the heart's blood supply they are extra susceptible to poor circulation. The common foot conditions that old people develop are corns and bunions, chilblains, ingrown toe nails and diseases of the skin such as dryness, cracking and even ulcers. Any of these may lead to an unpleasant infection. They can and should be prevented or at least dealt with as soon as they are noticed. Neglected feet are a source of great discomfort, and in cases that have been allowed to deteriorate badly will involve complicated medical treatment and even surgery. Old people with diabetes are especially at risk from infections. The importance of foot care is always emphasized to people with diabetes, but you should be especially vigilant if your relative has this condition.

In any case, reaching and caring for the feet is always hard for older people and leaving out that part of the washing routine is tempting. These suggestions should encourage proper foot care:

1. Wash the feet daily, and put on clean socks or stockings. Cut toe nails regularly.

2. Inspect the feet twice weekly, looking for discolorations, cracks between the toes, or blisters. Ask the chiropodist or doctor for advice and treatment if any of these occurs.

3. Corns and calluses should be treated by a chiropodist, especially when someone has diabetes. Hard skin should not be cut at with a razor, or other instrument.

4. Avoid causing any break in the skin, and infection. Never apply strong antiseptics. Do not use corn plasters or commercial corn cures, as they too may cause skin damage.

5. Circulation can be endangered by pressure, cold, smoking, sitting for long periods cross-legged, wearing socks with elastic tops, and sometimes wading or bathing in cold water.

6. Do not put the feet in hot water without first testing to see if the temperature is between 85 and 90°F (30 and 32°C), or warm them in front of direct heat. This may cause painful eruptions and cracked skin.

7. Always wear comfortable, well-fitting shoes with good support. When buying a new pair, choose carefully, as late in the day as possible. The feet swell gradually, and shoes bought in the morning may pinch by the late afternoon.

8. Walking is the best exercise for the feet and promotes good circulation.

We have tried in this chapter to give some guidance on recognizing and treating the minor ailments and discomforts of old age. Another aspect of caring is to preserve what health remains, and with your relative living under the same roof you will be able to have more influence on this positive side of health care.

Maintaining good health

When asked their secret of a long and healthy life old people give answers that are often contradictory. To some it comes from quiet contentment, to others from constant challenge and variety; some eat a lot, some little; some eat meat, others are vegetarians. Whatever the reasons an old person gives, your concern is to be able to recognize and maintain a state of good health.

This requires some experience. Even when an old person declares that he feels fine, we must allow ourselves a certain amount of scepticism, because there is often a reluctance to admit to feeling unwell. Appearances may be deceptive, simply because some people's skin becomes paler and more sallow, while in others the tiny blood vessels enlarge, giving what seems like a healthy glow. So, how can you make an accurate estimate? Here are two useful indications:

1. How energetic is your relative? It is a reasonable yardstick to assume that people who have the energy to do all they want are in good health. You can obtain a fair impression by watching and

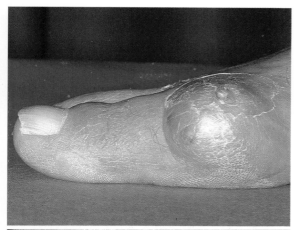

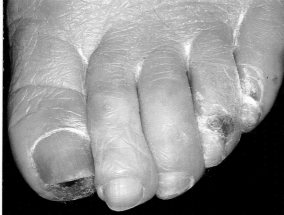

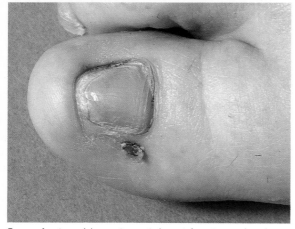

Some foot problems to watch out for: *top*, a bunion, *centre*, ulcers on the toes and, *bottom*, an ingrowing toenail.

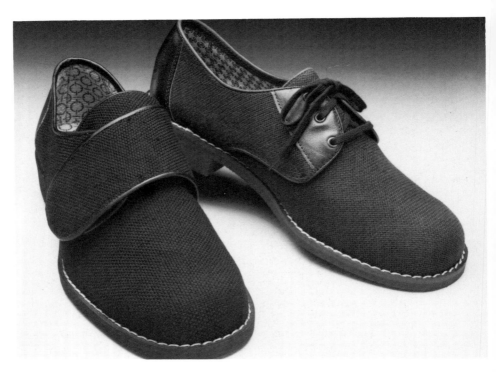

There are now special shoes for people with problem feet in many different styles.

listening for lively speech and gestures during ordinary conversation.

2. How interested is your relative in what is going on, and in planning ahead? Healthy people are optimistic and outward-looking with a willingness to devote themselves to larger interests, despite the odd ache or pain.

Most old people are concerned about maintaining good health, and are glad to discuss various ways of making improvements. On the other hand, they are conservative and do not welcome great changes being imposed on their lifestyle. By far the best way is to talk simply about the advantages and disadvantages of new ways, and to be sympathetic. After all, none of us likes changing our ways without very good reason. It is fruitless to be impatient with someone who will not take good advice. When unwelcome suggestions have to be made they may come best from a professional person, such as your family doctor.

Ways to preserve good health
Eating   This is basic to maintaining good health. Enjoying food is a continuing pleasure throughout life. But some old people are difficult

about food, and others may even be undernourished. This may be due to depression and isolation, or to poverty. Others are unable to go out shopping and will make do with anything at hand. Then there are those who have never been very skilled cooks and have now perhaps become confused. Finally, some become food faddists and restrict their intake to a narrow range of foods, perhaps through having misunderstood medical advice about diet. Poor appetite can of course be a feature of gastrointestinal disease, and if your relative stops eating properly you will have to use your judgment as to whether this is the reason.

An obese elderly person will need to reduce the intake of high-energy foods such as fats and refined sugar, for carrying excess weight makes the development of diabetes, arthritis and diseases of the heart and blood vessels more likely.

How much should your relative eat?　It is best for an older person to have small meals frequently. This is easier on the digestion and maintains a regular energy level. Despite the comments above, older people do not need a lot of food, and you shouldn't worry if your relative has a small appetite. However, a few guidelines on the ideal type of diet should be useful.

The best foods for most older people are the same as for anyone else – low in sugar and fat, but high in roughage, fresh vegetables and fruit, with 2 oz (50 g) of protein in the form of meat, fish or eggs, low-fat milk or cheese. Obviously, for anyone with diverticular disease or a condition such as diabetes, the fibre and fat content will have to be adjusted following medical advice.

In general, food should be fresh rather than processed. A frequent helping of raw foods such as grated vegetables provides full nutritional value as well as ensuring an intake of roughage, essential for healthy bowel opening. For the same reasons wholegrain bread and brown rice are better than white. Calcium is needed to maintain an aging person's bone strength. The recommended daily intake is 800–1000 mg per day. This can be taken as a pint of low-fat milk, or 1 oz (25 g) of cheese. But calcium is also present in some vegetables (see the table, page 48), and it can be taken in tablet form. Since a reduction in the saturated fats found especially in animal products is now generally recommended, it is best to boost calcium intake with this variety of foods.

Beef, pork and lamb all contain more than 20 per cent fat even in lean slices, so that chicken (with 3.4 per cent fat) and turkey (with 1.7 per cent fat) are better. It is not often realized that, as a bonus, chicken is richer in iron than steak! Any added fat should be restricted, but is better in the form of polyunsaturated margarine rather than butter. The added vitamin D in margarine is also good for old people. Sunflower, safflower and olive oils are recommended for cooking by nutritionists.

Ways of increasing calcium intake

Calcium content of pills available over the counter

	Pills providing 600 mg
Calcium gluconate 600 mg contains 54 mg calcium	12
Calcium lactate 300 mg contains 44 mg calcium	14
Sandocal – 4.5 g contains 400 mg calcium	1½

Calcium content of common foods in mg per 100 g (3½ oz approx) of food

Dairy

	mg
Cheese	
Cheddar	800
Cottage (low fat soft cheese)	60
Danish Blue	580
Edam	740
Parmesan	1220
processed	700
spread	510
Cream	79
Egg (whole)	52
Egg (yolk)	130
Milk (3.53 fl oz/98 ml)	120
Yoghurt – low fat (5 oz/145 ml)	180

Meat and fish

Meat contains very small amounts of calcium, as does fish.
Meat pies and fish in batter contain calcium in the flour.
Canned pilchards and sardines, sprats and whitebait contain calcium in the bones.

	mg
Boiled prawns	150
Canned crab	120
pilchards	300
salmon	93
sardines	460–550
Fried sprats	620–710
whitebait	860
Fish paste	280
Steamed scallops	120

Vegetables

	mg
Beans, haricot (navy)	180
kidney	140
Broccoli	100
Cabbage	53
Chick peas (garbanzos)	140
Greens, turnip, cale, collard, mustard	98
Olives in brine	61
Parsley	330
Peas (boiled/frozen)	31
Spinach (boiled)	600
Spring onions (scallions)	140
Watercress	220

Fruit

	mg
Apricots, dried	82
Blackcurrants, raw	60
Currants, dried	95
Figs, dried	280
Lemon, whole	110
Rhubarb, raw	100

Nuts (shelled weight)

Almonds	250
Barcelonas	170
Brazils	180
Peanuts (groundnuts), roasted and salted	61
Sesame seeds	870

Drinks (dry weight)

Cocoa powder	130
Coffee, ground	130
instant	160
Malted milk drink (Horlicks)	230
Tea, India	430

Cooking ingredients

Baking powder (depending on brand)	11300
Curry powder	640
Mustard, dry	330
Pepper	130
Salt, block	230
Stock cubes (depending on brand)	180
Yeast, dried	80

Flour and baked foods

Bread (white or brown)	100
Hovis (UK)	150
Cake, sponge (fatless)	140
rock (individual fruit cakes)	390
Flour, plain (cake)	130
self-raising	350
Soya flour	210–40
Wheat bran	110

Salt is now considered to be a factor in increasing high blood pressure. Many old people suffer from this condition, so should eat less salt. It is probably a good idea for everyone to cut down on salt intake. In any case, food tastes fresher and more appetizing once you have become used to the blander flavours (see *The Salt-Free Diet Book* by Dr Graham MacGregor, in this series).

Old people often have sweet foods and candies around and eat them regularly throughout the day. For obvious reasons – especially to avoid putting on weight and increasing tooth decay – these should be eaten sparingly. Nevertheless, a little extra sugar can give a necessary spurt of energy to an old person who is feeling fatigued, so sweets need not be entirely excluded, except for people with diabetes.

A diet containing the right ingredients needs no supplementation. The enjoyment of a wide range of fresh foods ensures an adequate intake of vitamins. A course of vitamin B_{12} or vitamin C may be recommended by your doctor for specific deficiencies, but it is unwise to take these without medical advice. One vitamin, though, does need watching. This is vitamin D, which, being produced under the skin through the action of sunlight, might be considered to be more of a hormone. It is essential for maintaining minerals such as calcium and phosphorus in bone. In countries where during the winter months the amount of sunlight is limited, it is important to encourage sufficient exposure to the sun's rays during the summer for enough vitamin D to be stored. Even in countries that enjoy year round sunshine, old people are inclined to cover up. Too much exposure brings the danger of skin cancer, but thirty minutes in the sun, as long as it's not at a time when the rays are harmful, builds up the vitamin D stores effectively. Dietary supplements of vitamin D are helpful, but less effective.

What about drinks? The body requires at least three pints (1.5 litres) of liquid each day to enable the kidneys to clear waste products from the system. But even for an invalid I would not recommend those expensive but fattening tinted drinks containing gas and glucose. Fresh fruit drinks, and canned and frozen ones, low-fat milk and tea or coffee in moderation are usually suitable.

Alcohol Taking small quantities of the weaker alcoholic drinks such as a glass of beer or wine with a meal is pleasurable and encourages relaxed enjoyment, but drinking hard spirits should be limited. Having a glass of spirits to 'keep out the cold' is most unwise, and a fallacy, since the sensation of warmth is due to opening up the skin vessels to carry more blood, resulting in rapid heat loss. It is never a good idea to have an alcoholic drink at bedtime. Although this may induce sleep to start with, it also produces restlessness, and a desire to pass urine more frequently.

Smoking is now well known to be a major contributor to the development of lung cancer, and even more so of heart disease, and should be discouraged. It can reduce the appetite, blunt the sense of taste and smell, cause bad breath and indigestion, and alter the normal rhythm of the heartbeat.

There is also the attendant danger of fire to consider. Old people can easily fall asleep before extinguishing a cigarette butt.

Drugs Many old people take medicines regularly. Do not be surprised if you find your relative is taking a selection of drugs, or not taking drugs that have been prescribed. Although most doctors do their best to help older people comply with their treatment, you may find that the whole business has become chaotic. One reason for this is that for each new illness there is a treatment, which tends to be taken even after the symptoms have stopped. Geriatricians frequently point out the hazards of polypharmacy, but I have always marvelled at how old people are able to tolerate so many different drugs at the same time.

I suggest that you ask your doctor to assess your relative's medication when you begin caring for him or her. You should ensure that the prescribed drugs are taken at their recommended times. Many have been formulated for slow release, to be taken once daily. Of course, this means remembering the single dose is very important. It should not take long to establish a routine.

If your relative prefers taking liquid preparations to pills or capsules, which have been prescribed, don't try and buy an alternative medicine without advice. Solid tablets can be crushed into a powder and taken in water or in a spoonful of jam.

It will be up to you to notice the effects of drugs on your relative. Side effects can result from taking almost any drug, and may affect people in different ways. Signs to watch for are: skin rashes, dry mouth, visual disturbances, nausea and vomiting, feeling faint, bladder disturbance, mental changes and jaundice. The more drugs taken at any one time, the greater the risk of side effects developing. One way of telling which drug is responsible is to withhold the suspected one for a few days, and then to give it again, but this should not be done without first consulting with the doctor.

If the relative you are caring for is still living away from you, it is helpful to draw up a weekly chart, and the times marked on each day when the different drugs are to be taken. Check that your relative is able to use this memory aid; otherwise you will need to give the medicines and mark the chart yourself when you visit.

Exercise It is important that your relative maintains a lifestyle that includes the right amount of exercise. This strengthens the heart through increasing the circulation of the blood, and brings additional benefits – better muscle tone, enhanced appetite, regular bowel function and a greater sense of wellbeing. With exercise, more oxygen is

50

taken into the blood. As the heart begins to receive more blood from the veins its muscle fibres are stretched out, and it beats more forcefully and rapidly. Small blood vessels, many of which are closed during inactivity, begin to open and allow blood to flow and nourish the tissues.

Since the body's reserves of energy are reduced with age, there are limits to the amount of exercise that can be taken by old people. For them daily routine chores provide a large amount of what is required and it is unwise for them to try violent, sudden or prolonged exercise. Better to wait for the next bus than to run for this one! An older person who is unaccustomed to exercise can quickly feel fatigued because the heart is unable to cope with the extra demand. Very often there are warnings that the danger limits are being approached, such as pain in the chest or shortness of breath. Exercise should not be taken beyond the point where tiredness begins. When any of the above signs appear, tell your relative to sit and relax, and breathe deeply. Report any further symptoms to your doctor.

Of the various forms of exercise, walking is the easiest and one of the most beneficial, being rhythmical and moderate in its demands. But for those accustomed to it, swimming is excellent exercise, so is dancing, and many older people continue to play golf and tennis, to ride a bicycle and do gardening.

Some exercise can be taken indoors, and a programme of limb stretching and putting all the joints through a full range of movement is an ideal way of exercising whatever your capabilities or limitations. The routine should be regular, and with practice can be extended and built up (see the suggestions on page 52).

However, many older people are handicapped and any exercise is difficult. What is not good is sitting for long periods with the knees bent, weakening the thigh muscles. Chairbound people with a little mobility should put their legs out straight, and lift them towards the ceiling from time to time. The old rocking chair is a good way of exercising the legs without putting the whole of the body weight on them.

Sex Some people think that it is inappropriate, even indecent, if not outrageous, for an older person to have sexual feelings. Others think that it is dangerous to continue sexual activity in later life. On the contrary, the expression of sexual feeling between two older people is a sign of health. I have encountered old men staying with well-meaning children who have understood their every want except sexual fulfilment. It is a widely held myth that the elderly are asexual, and children seem to have a natural reluctance to look upon a parent's sexual aspirations as wholesome. The truth is that warm affection and its physical expression are even more highly prized among the elderly, for whom opportunity is more restricted, than in younger people.

A daily exercise sequency. Repeat 4 times on each side, building up gradually to 16.

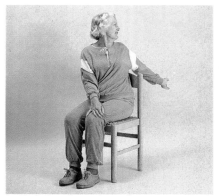 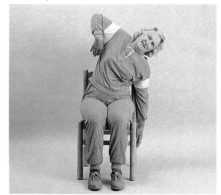

1. Twisting from the spine, use your arm as a lever to further movement, and follow through with your head erect.
2. Side bend as far as you can and feel the stretch up the side of your body, relaxing your neck and taking the head over with the spine.

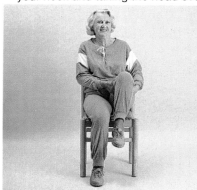 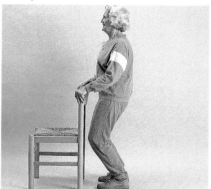

3. Lift your leg from under your thigh as high as possible, maintaining good posture.
4. Bend and straighten, keeping your back straight, abdomen contracted and seat pulled under. Progress to rising gently on your toes and lowering again when you've mastered this one.

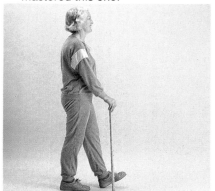 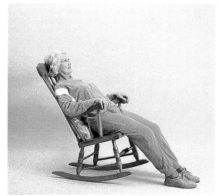

5. Draw yourself up to your full height, pulling in your abdomen and behind and straightening your legs. Walk from heel to toe, using the stick for support.
6. Push right back in the chair to get a full stretch on the thigh muscles.

Mental activity and stimulation Throughout life the mind needs stimulation, much as the body needs food and exercise. Some people who are by nature solitary and lead an energetic mental life, reading or listening to the radio, seem to have little need of others. Most of us, however, are dependent on the stimulation derived from conversation, both to maintain mental agility and to prevent ideas becoming fixed and attitudes hardened. The natural place for conversation is in the home, but with television becoming more popular every day, the old art of conversing is taking second place.

As the years pass we have to face the fact that some close relatives and friends will die at a time when we are most dependent on them, and it is not easy when one is older to make new friends to fill the gaps. So is it not important to maintain friendships we have made, in spite of the effort needed to get out and meet friends, and of the effects of age and illness on the personality, which can lead to displays of ill-nature or self-centredness?

Bodily disorders focus attention on self, and can prevent enjoyment of outside interests, friends and family. Yet a mind that is not fed can become dulled or disordered, so you should encourage as much stimulation as you can.

Membership of special interest clubs or societies affords the opportunity to meet and communicate with others of all ages. In this way new friendships are made. Our contribution is to see that elderly people do

Day clubs are ideal for making friends and taking up new interests.

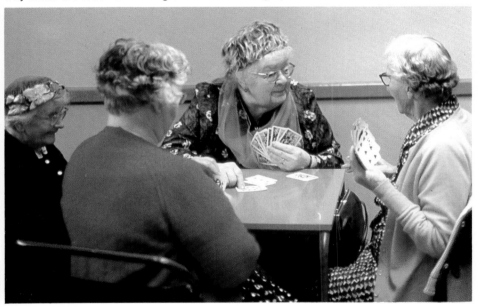

not always reminisce about the past, but are encouraged to discuss their future plans and development. They should be able to talk about their interests, and it is important to ask their opinion, but not to patronize them so that they can get away with statements without being challenged. By expecting old people to 'be their age' – whatever that means – we are responsible for moulding them into has-beens.

For those never prepared for old age, the compulsorily retired and those of incomplete education, keeping interests alive is often especially difficult. But it is not impossible to acquire the habit of mental work in old age, and much of the excitement of later life is in learning new things. I shall never forget meeting my sister-in-law off the boat from Brazil, when she told us that she had heard an old lady broadcasting there on the Overseas Service in Portuguese. She was ninety and had learned the language during the past three years, and had passed the advanced examination. By coincidence, we knew this lady, and I remember meeting her two years later, when she was ninety-two, sitting on a bench in the centre of our town slumped in depression because she had learned that day that she had failed an examination in religious studies.

The mind is fed also by the use of the hands, and this is the basis of occupational therapy. Many old people who have never had time to indulge an artistic talent discover an ability to paint or draw in advanced age. Not everyone will become a Grandma Moses, but that does not matter, so long as the mind is stimulated and activity retained.

Prestige and the retention of personality
We have already discussed your adjusting relationship in Chapter 2. But certain aspects have a strong bearing on a healthy body and mind. When an elderly person leaves home to live with someone else there is a period of mutual adjustment. You and your elderly relative have developed along very different lines over a long span of years. The relationship began a long time ago, and much of the colouring of those days will be brought back to mind. However, that old relationship now has no part to play. The parental role should have finished when you became an adult. There should be affectionate friendship, and the better part of a love in which you hold each other in mutual respect.

I do not say that relationships are easily managed, but I do suggest how we might aim to establish them. The mistakes are made by attempting to rekindle or continue an outmoded bond, instead of beginning afresh and creating a new, living relationship from the old foundations, therefore completing the structure.

4 PRACTICAL NURSING

Even old people's illnesses are usually minor, and they have good chances of recovery. Few require admission to the hospital. But elderly people are more vunerable to colds and influenza and need careful attention so that complications don't develop. Nursing a sick relative at home falls mainly on companions and relations. Usually home nursing requires no more than basic common sense and physical fitness. Only in more complicated or chronic illnesses may a trained nurse be needed. Nursing has traditionally been a woman's task, but men can also nurse with strength, skill and compassion. In this chapter I give some practical advice on caring for your relative during illness and disability.

The most common reasons for being confined to bed are a chest infection, influenza, a minor case of heart failure or a gastric upset. For any of these you will have to nurse an elderly person for a week or two. Longer periods in bed are undesirable.

The role of the family doctor is important. It is he or she who makes the diagnosis and the assessment for treatment. Since old people tend to suffer not from one but from a collection of illnesses and disabilities, nursing involves a lot more than just taking drugs and medicines. Your doctor will also be able to give some idea of the course the illness might take, and how long it will last. This is called the prognosis. It can of course only be an educated guess, but it is of great importance when you are considering your resources, and your other commitments.

What care can you provide?
Your first aim must be your relative's comfort. You can best achieve this with sensitivity and considering such straightforward matters as cleanliness, warmth, nourishment and rest. Information about special equipment will be useful and the best way of finding out what is available is to ask your doctor. Among the aids that help the bedridden there are padded footrests placed at the foot of the bed that prevent the patient slipping down, backrests that stop pillows from slipping when the patient is seated in bed and sheepskin pads to prevent bed sores. Most home nursing equipment can be rented or loaned from nursing stores, social services departments, or the Red Cross (see Chapter 9).

The second objective is to prevent complications such as congestion of the lungs, pressure sores or depression by devising a programme of physical and mental activity. This should begin as soon as your relative

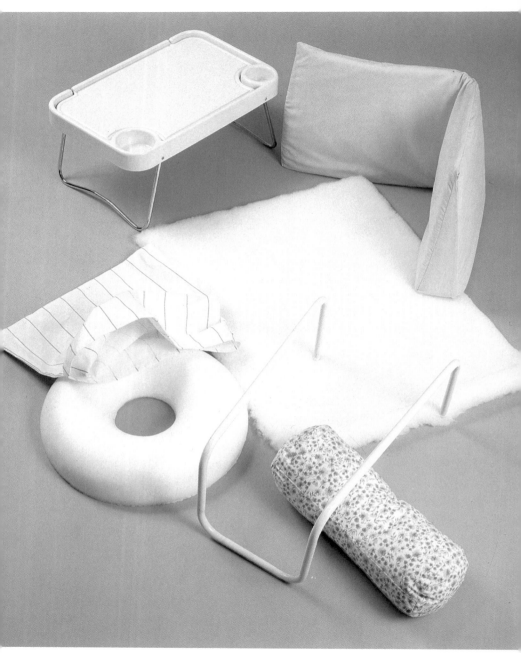

Home nursing aids (clockwise): a bed tray that can be adjusted to hold a book; a hinged cushion for support while sitting up in bed; a sheepskin pad to prevent pressure sores; a metal frame to keep heavy bedclothes off the legs; a neck cushion; and a ring cushion.

is fit to leave bed. Whenever possible he or she should wear normal day clothes as this has an important positive psychological effect. While sitting out of bed the invalid should do stretching and deep breathing exercises. Not only will this provide exercise and improve circulation, but it will also encourage independence.

Apart from these physical aspects, you must be able to reassure and set your relative on the road to recovery. You have to be firm yet tactful about persuading your relative to get up, and be prepared sometimes for accusations of unkindness. The fact is that bed is a dangerous place, as we shall see later. Besides, sitting out of bed makes reading, talking to visitors, doing jigsaw puzzles, playing card games or writing letters easier. It is also more comfortable to eat sitting in a chair, with suitable support.

Finally, you need to preserve and increase mental independence and confidence. Try to make your relative take responsibility as much as possible for his or her affairs, and deal with correspondence. Motivation is a valuable ally in the fight against illness.

The sick room

You may have already adapted your relative's bedroom along the lines I suggested in Chapter 2, so that it is suitable as a sick room. If your relative has been fit and able-bodied up till now, you will have to prepare a sick room, bearing the following points in mind:

1. Decide first where it should be. It will probably be a bedroom, unless all the bedrooms are situated too far for convenience – upstairs, for instance. This will impose a strain on the nurse, especially if she is not young, and may make communication difficult. Then, a room near where you are working and near the kitchen will have to be converted.

2. The sick room must be near the bathroom (see also Chapter 2).

3. It should be free of obstacles that restrict movement. But do provide a comfortable armchair for your relative to sit in.

4. The temperature should be maintained at between 68 and 72°F (20 and 22°C), with good ventilation.

The bed

If possible, place the bed near a window for good light and ventilation, and with access to your relative's right-hand side so that he or she can be lifted and turned. The bed should be on castors so it is mobile, and wide enough to avoid the danger of falling out due to restlessness. The height of the bed is important. From the nurse's point of view a higher bed is best because it does not call for arduous bending. If, on the other

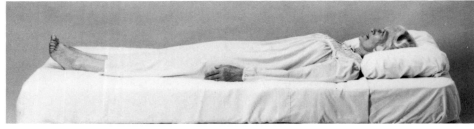

Exercises for the bedridden:
1. Lie as flat as you can, contracting your thigh and seat muscles. Push your abdominal muscles towards the bed and obliquely under the ribs. Tense the muscles and relax several times.

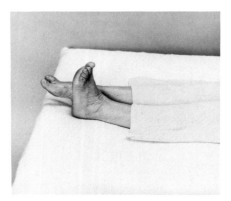

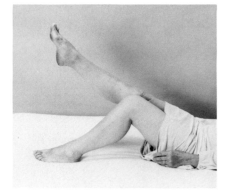

2. Point your feet alternately to floor and ceiling 4–16 times to mobilize your ankles and strengthen your legs.

3. Straighten each knee and bend down 4 times to strengthen the calves and thighs.

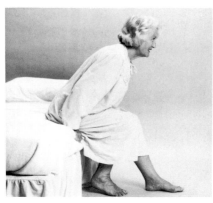

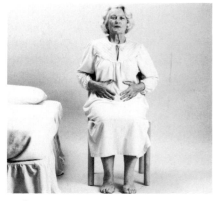

4. Getting up from the bed, place one foot well in front of the other, lean forward, and bracing your arms, push up well with the back foot. Done several times this is also a good exercise for the legs.

5. Sit erect, breathe deeply and slowly, to expand the lungs. Inhale through your nose and exhale through your mouth to your fullest extent, without force.

Note When you are no longer in bed, combine these exercises with the sequence on page 52 to give your body a good workout.

hand, the patient is restless or confused a higher bed is a potential hazard. The mattress should be firm unless your relative will be bed-ridden for a long time (see page 67).

Bedclothing should be lightweight, and not tucked in tightly, especially over the feet – for those who are used to them, lightweight comforters or quilts suit very well. A metal frame placed over the feet will allow full movement. If your relative complains of cold feet, provide bedsocks. These are preferable to hot water bottles, which may burn and are any-way only a temporary source of warmth, and to electric blankets as they do not supply direct heat to the feet. The safest position is to sit up against a prop of pillows supported by a backrest. This eases breathing and avoids congestion of the lungs. While your relative has to be in bed, encourage exercising the ankles and calf muscles and hourly deep breathing exercises.

Clothing should be light and loose, without constriction around the neck or limbs. While your relative needs constant nursing, a large nightshirt which opens up behind and is loosely tied together with tapes may be the most practical garment. In any case, cotton nightwear is

Sitting up in bed: for good support, make a prop of at least three pillows, one at the base with two crossed over it.

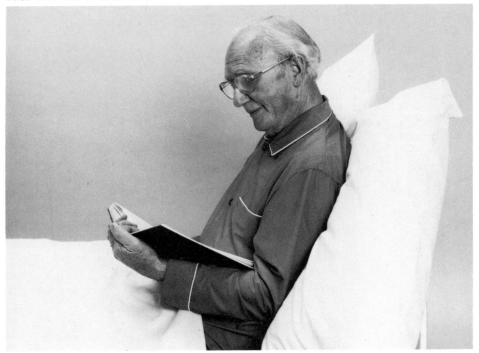

more comfortable than nylon. As many older people feel cold around the shoulders after sitting in bed for any length of time, have a shawl or bedjacket available for sitting up.

The dangers of bed

I have already mentioned the dangers of allowing a sick person to stay too long in bed. Elderly people must get up as long as they are able.

- Sitting up in bed for long periods creates pressure on the lower spine leading to back problems and the dangers of bed sores (see page 66).
- Sitting in bed, the calf muscles are not contracted, so that the blood is pooled in the veins, causing a danger of thrombosis.
- Unused muscles begin to waste, losing bulk and strength, so that an old person kept in bed finds it difficult to walk.
- There is also the danger of contracture. The weight of the bed-clothes on the feet extends the ankle into a position where the foot is dropped.
- Most people kept in bed become depressed and withdrawn, enveloped by the invalid state.

If you are unsure whether it is safe to allow your relative out of bed, ask your doctor's advice. My rule is that anyone who is ill should be allowed out of bed for at least part of the day. Only someone in the terminal stages of an illness will not be able to get up.

Practical nursing

How much can you do? For everyday nursing such as washing and feeding you don't need training. Common sense and the advice your doctor gives you as well as the hints in this book will see you through minor illness or disablement. For serious cases you will need the assistance of a trained nurse and of course this will be arranged through your doctor. These are the daily tasks that will be necessary when your relative is ill:

Washing and cleanliness   At least once a day your relative should have an all-over wash. There is no problem if he or she can get to a washbasin or can wash himself in bed. The illustrations opposite show how you can give a bed bath if neither of these is possible. This is a matter of working systematically in such a way that the sick person does not get cold. Areas requiring special attention are the buttocks, the genital region and under the breasts.

Cleaning the teeth regularly both helps prevent decay and makes the mouth feel fresh, especially when people are reluctant to drink. Rinsing

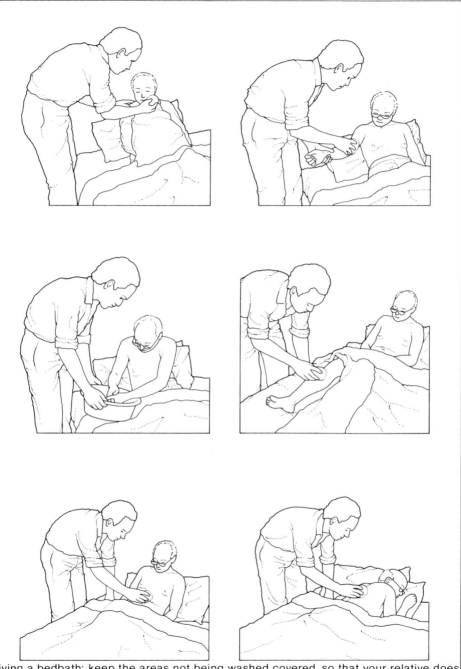

Giving a bedbath: keep the areas not being washed covered, so that your relative does not become cold.

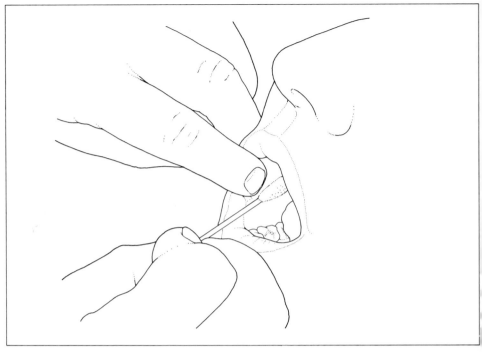

Cleaning an old person's mouth with a moist cotton wool swab; alternatively, use gauze wrapped around your index finger.

with a suitable mouthwash after meals is a good idea, but if this isn't possible, you can clean the mouth with a piece of surgical gauze moistened in water and wrapped around a clean small stick or your index finger.

The difficulties that used to be encountered with shaving an old man have disappeared since electric razors came into use.

After the main daily wash, it gives a great boost to groom the nails and the hair. Elderly ladies appreciate having a cologne or cologne stick for occasional freshening, though without an overpowering scent.

Eating For guidelines on the type of food that is appropriate for old people, see Chapter 3. 'Invalid' foods are no longer considered necessary, though you will have to cater for a diminished appetite during illness by adapting the normal diet, and you should first consult your doctor about any special needs. You will also have to make sure your relative can chew and digest easily. If chewing is difficult the food will have to be minced. Or using two hands may not be possible; then you can provide a plate that is fixed in position and fitted with a rim to prevent the food being pushed over. Much help in these matters is obtainable from a handicapped resource centre (see Chapter 9).

Lifting Inevitably the sick person will need to be lifted many times a day, to be helped on to a bedpan, or after slipping down, or simply to be made more comfortable. This can be difficult for an inexperienced person, and you should try to get someone to help: you link hands across the bed. The linked arms are placed under the sick person's thighs, and the lift is made by a concerted movement (see the photographs on page 64). Although singlehanded lifting is not desirable, there is often no alternative. Here is a safe method:

1. To avoid injuring your back, always bend your knees and keep your back straight.
2. Most ill people are capable of understanding and can help by bending their knees, digging in with their heels.
3. The very ill or semi-conscious patient will be unable to do this. You should place your right knee on the bed up by the right hip and steady yourself by grasping the back of the bed with your left arm. By this means you should be able to lift your patient from under the armpit.

   Alternatively, you can bring the patient's legs over the side of

A rimmed plate held in place with a rubber mat makes eating with only one hand easy.

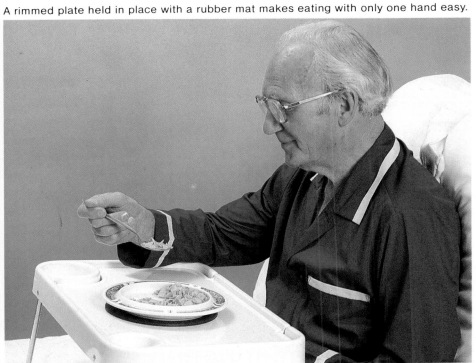

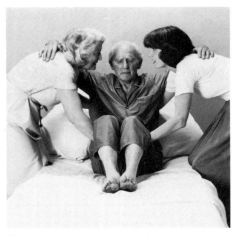

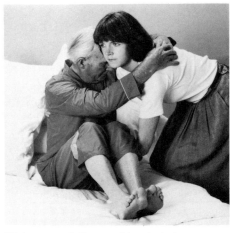

Ways of moving your relative in bed:

With two people, link hands under the thighs and across the lower back

With your relative pushing to help

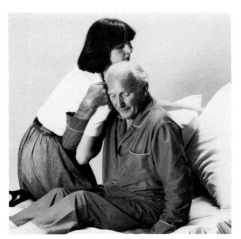

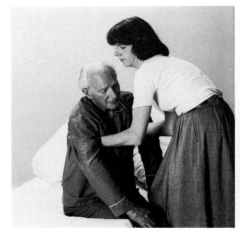

Using your knee for extra purchase, lift very gently under the armpit not to damage delicate nerves. Never lift someone who has had a stroke and is paralysed on that side.

An easier way may be to 'sit' the patient along the bed.

the bed to face you, and then grasp him under the armpits and shift him a few inches, repeating a few times if necessary before you lift his legs back into the bed.

Excretions   The home nurse must have a policy for dealing with the actions of bowel and bladder. This is a very intimate and personal matter, and one which is perhaps even more embarrassing for the patient. So it is best to bring the matter out into the open – and not to forget your sense of humour should things go wrong.

Many old people become anxious about moving their bowels, especially when there is nothing to pass. Naturally, this happens when there has been little or no food eaten, and you can give reassurance that there is nothing to worry about. There is, though, a possibility of constipation after an inactive period on a bland, restricted diet, so it is important to find out what the regular rhythm is (see Chapter 3).

Whenever possible your relative should be encouraged to go to the toilet: even very frail people prefer to be helped out of bed rather than offered a bedpan. If the distance is too great, a commode can be an invaluable alternative and it may also be used as a chair for sitting out of

To give a bedpan lift your relative with one arm and slide the pan underneath. *Right* The arms are straight for support and the knees very slightly bent.

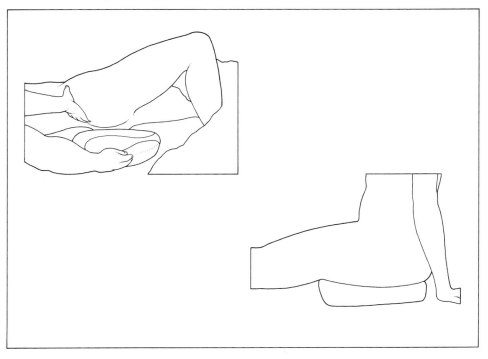

bed. It is particularly useful for women with restricted mobility who need to pass urine fairly frequently. Most men can manage to pass urine into a urine bottle.

Difficulty with sleeping Sleep disturbance happens with sick people because of physical or mental discomfort. Using sedatives to alleviate them can make things worse. Physical causes are due to:

- Pain, resulting from indigestion, or from arthritic pain when turning over
- Breathlessness
- Nausea
- Skin irritation.

All these may be brought on by a condition you already know about, or may signal the start of an illness. It is important to note where and when they occur, how long they last and what relieves them, to help later diagnosis.

Mental causes of sleeplessness are:

- Worry from a feeling of being alone or due to overactivity of the imagination
- Worry that not sleeping itself will make the illness worse
- Nightmares, confusion on waking at night, may be caused by infection or by prescribed drugs.

The last will need the doctor's advice. Otherwise mental discomfort may be alleviated by the considerate treatment I describe in Chapter 3. I do not usually recommend sedatives during illness, or at any other time. These are not really good for old people and may cause unsteadiness if they rise at night, or produce hangover effects throughout the day. Nevertheless, when someone has been taking sleeping pills for some time without harmful effects, it is probably as well to continue with them while sleeplessness is especially likely.

Special problems
Pressure sores, or bed sores These are a very real danger for elderly people who spend a long time in bed. They can develop into unpleasant wounds so must be avoided at all costs. They appear where there are bony protruberances, for example, at the lower back, elbows, knees and heels, when the blood supply is restricted after long periods of lying or sitting. The old idea of rubbing the areas with soap and water and then rubbing in alcohol has no effect. The bedridden person must be told to move into different positions at least every hour, or if very weak, you have to move him or her.

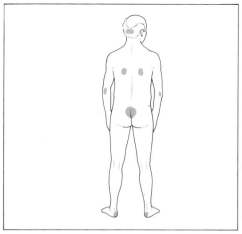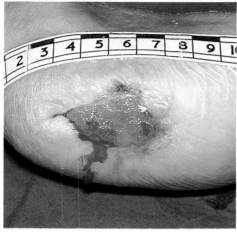

Left The red areas show where pressure sores are most likely to occur. *Right* A sore that has been neglected can become a nasty wound.

If your relative finds movement difficult, it is advisable to borrow or invest in a ripple mattress at the outset. These mattresses produce a series of pressure changes which prevent any one part from being subjected to undue pressure for long. Air-filled ring cushions and sheepskin or foam pads for the heels and elbows are also useful aids.

Bed sores cannot always be avoided. The first sign is for the skin over the susceptible parts to become dry and red. As soon as you see any sign of this you should speak to your doctor or the nurse attending your relative.

Other points to remember when nursing a sick person are:

1. Give all prescribed medicines correctly at the right times.
2. Special precautions during infectious illness:
   - Arrange for a separate room.
   - Do not allow visitors, animals or pets.
   - Put on a clean gown to nurse your relative, and keep it hanging inside the sick room.
   - Wash your hands before putting on the gown and after nursing.
   - Keep the invalid's dishes separate from everyone else's. Wash them in detergent after a ten-minute soak in boiling water, and then rinse. Disposable paper dishes are a convenient alternative.

- Collect the bed linen in a disposable plastic bag, soak in disinfectant and launder separately in the hottest possible wash.
- Final cleaning of the sickroom after your relative has recovered is important. Seek advice from your doctor about the need for either disinfection or fumigation.

Hints on nursing the common disorders

We have already seen in this chapter how certain illnesses are common enough to be expected in anyone over seventy. Here I describe in a little more detail those common conditions that do not demand hospitalization, or even a prolonged time in bed at home. But your relative will need careful monitoring and reminding to follow the doctor's advice on medical treatment and lifestyle.

Heart disease

Heart disease is common in old age. The failing heart is unable to pump blood efficiently around the body's network of arteries, either because of changes that take place in the pumping muscle, or because the heart cannot push blood against the pressure set up in the miles of blood vessels. Then again the heart may beat unevenly, causing tiredness and shortness of breath. Some people with heart disease feel pain when they make a physical effort or become emotional. This is felt in the centre of the chest and may radiate across and down the arm. The pain is called angina.

Heart disease can now be markedly relieved by modern treatment, so that people survive for many years. New drugs to lower pressure, increase pumping efficiency and improve heart rhythms are prescribed. Surgical treatment such as installing pacemakers and replacing narrowed blood vessels are commonplace.

Home care

1. The tendency seems to be to do everything to make an elderly heart patient as active as possible, even including undertaking vigorous exercise. Yet there is something to be said for the old-fashioned treatment of seating the invalid in a rocking chair with a blanket round the knees. Both methods have their place, and you have to learn, with advice from your doctor and by experience, when rest is advisable.

2. The only time the heart has to rest is between contractions, and when the pulse rate is advanced there is very little rest for the heart muscle. During sleep the rate drops, hence the need for regular hours of sleep. Since breathlessness is a normal feature it is better to arrange for the daytime rest in a chair – lying flat in bed is uncomfortable and piled up pillows often do not give enough support.

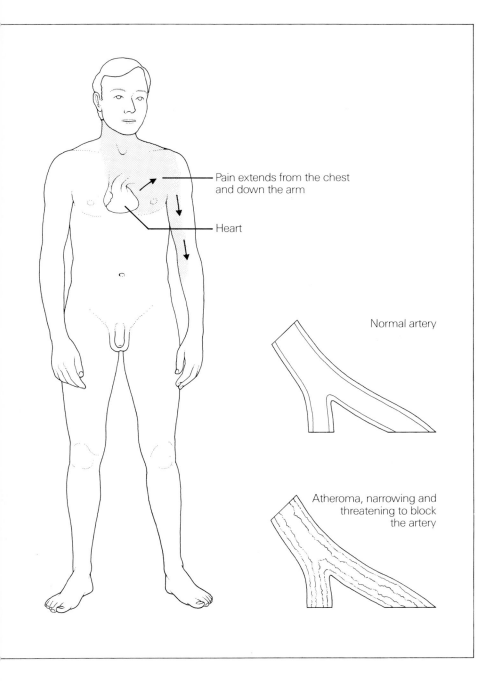

Pain extends from the chest
and down the arm

Heart

Normal artery

Atheroma, narrowing and
threatening to block
the artery

Coronary heart disease is caused by the arteries narrowing so the blood supply is
reduced, resulting in angina. A clot is also more likely to form on the irregular lining of
the arteries.

3. You should always try to avoid anxiety and any emotional upset which may cause the heart to react, such as taking your relative in the car during the rush hour.

4. Although it is difficult to remove excess weight in old age, especially when people cannot take sustained vigorous exercise, keeping to a low-fat and low-calorie, largely fresh vegetable diet is important. Even though this may not produce a big loss, it will prevent an increase in weight, as well as reduce the dangers of clogging the arteries and advancing the heart condition.

5. Swelling of the ankles and legs (dropsy or oedema) is often caused by the heart being unable to cope efficiently with pumping blood, due to congestion, so that excess fluid collects at the lower extremities. Diuretic pills are given to increase the amount of urine passed. Make sure they are taken regularly if prescribed for your relative.

A heart attack appears different from heart disease, being a sudden and dramatic event. This is due to a blockage (thrombosis) in one of the

Feet can swell up like this with heart disease. Note too how elderly people can neglect their feet when bending is hard.

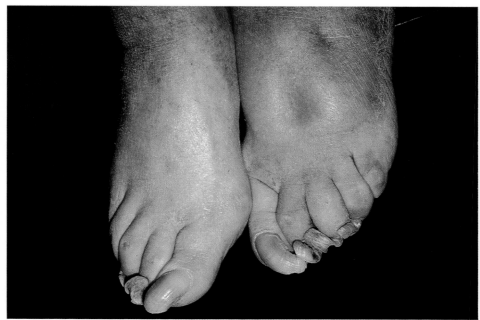

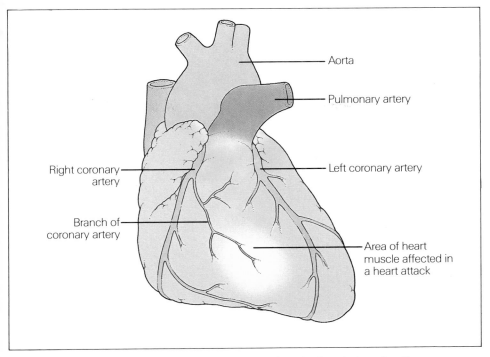

Aorta

Pulmonary artery

Right coronary artery

Left coronary artery

Branch of coronary artery

Area of heart muscle affected in a heart attack

A heart attack causes the muscle to seize up so that the heart stops beating.

arteries which supply the heart muscle, called the coronary arteries. The immediate signs may be pain in the chest, shock and pallor or mental confusion.

Heart attacks are common in the developed countries. They affect particularly middle-aged men and older women. Factors which make them more likely are being overweight, taking insufficient exercise, smoking and eating excessive quantities of animal fats. There is also more likelihood of an attack if another close member of the family is affected. Symptoms that should be regarded as warnings are:

- Unnatural tiredness
- Pains in the chest, arms and sometimes the neck and chin
- Shortness of breath
- Mental confusion.

Many people have angina (see above), and some may have it for years, knowing how to avoid it and when it will occur. This is called 'stable angina'. What is worrying, and the doctor should be consulted about it, is accelerating or crescendo angina, when the frequency and severity of pain increase.

The majority of older people's heart attacks are minor and the intensive care provided for a massive coronary thrombosis is not necessary. Your relative will be better off at home, in familiar surroundings, than in the hospital after a small heart attack. The journey can aggravate the attack, and 50 per cent of old people become confused when moved to the hospital suddenly. It is not necessary to stay in bed for more than a day or so. An old person's recovery is usually rather slow, with plenty of rest and slowly graded exercises needed for rehabilitation. These will be designed to be within the limits of your relative's tolerance, and you will have to encourage the progress towards better mobility.

Chest infections

Old people get chest infections especially in winter, and often without having a cold first. Those who suffer from chronic bronchitis or who smoke are particularly vulnerable. You will notice an increased rate of breathing and a bad cough, but your relative's temperature will not necessarily rise with a chest infection, as it does in younger people.

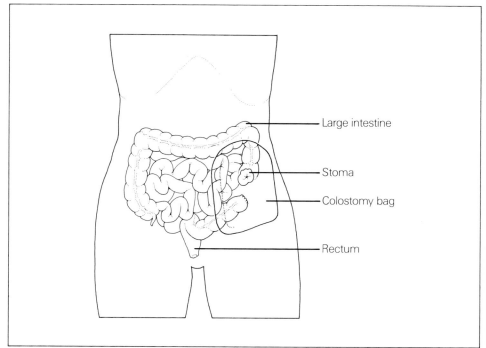

Colostomy: in this case part of the large intestine has been removed.

With people of advancing age the cough is weaker and less effective in bringing up phlegm, but if it is productive, your doctor will want to take a specimen for inspection.

Treatment of chest disorders with modern drugs is very effective, and the most suitable will be prescribed by your doctor. You can help in practical ways:

1. While your relative is in bed keep him or her propped up in the sitting position to make coughing and breathing easier.

2. Keep the room warm but well-ventilated.

3. Maintain the humidity at 50 per cent. In dry climates or with central heating use humidifiers in the room.

Colostomy

A colostomy or ileostomy operation is carried out to short cut a diseased length of the bowel due to cancer or chronic inflammation. The affected part is removed and an opening made in the abdominal wall to allow wastes to be passed out. The ileostomy is similar to the colostomy but a larger operation, which is not often performed on older people. Although not as common as the other conditions in this chapter, I feel colostomy is worth mentioning here because of the worry it can cause the elderly. People usually manage well and may have a normal life for many years. But it is difficult for an old person to cope for two reasons: mentally they are less flexible and so find it hard to adapt; and they usually lack manual dexterity and the ability to bend down and see for very long, so that dealing with the bag can be difficult.

Try and provide encouragement if your relative has to have this operation. The doctors and nurses will be very painstaking in teaching the skills needed for self-care, and with your help the situation will seem more acceptable. There are some famous people who have had this operation, who allow themselves to be quoted by the colostomy and ileostomy associations; and the many associations provide enormous support to colostomy patients.

5 THE MAJOR DISABILITIES OF OLD AGE

Illness is often difficult to understand in old people, not only by relatives and friends, but also by doctors. Whereas aging is clearly seen by others, illness is felt within. The aging process itself is adverse and relentless, but it is not a dustbin for throwing in every change noted in an old person. Appearances are very deceptive and in this and the next chapter we try to show how the four major disabilities of old age, with their multiple causes, themselves accumulate, eventually to become life-threatening to the elderly.

The features of illness in people over sixty are usually different from those among the younger groups. The start of an illness is often slow and insidious, and the symptoms do not conform to the usual descriptions. A mild heart attack may cause mental confusion rather than pain in the chest; or a thyroid condition, which would make a younger person overactive, can produce a state of fatigue and apathy in the elderly – so that illness is frequently mistaken for 'old age creeping on'. An illustration of this is the elderly person who begins a mysterious decline, and who, during observation and investigation in the hospital, recovers spontaneously.

There is often too a close relationship between physical illness and social conditions, so that nine out of ten elderly people who are admitted to the hospital or transferred to special homes are moved largely because of the breakdown of care at home. Old people tend to neglect their ailments for reasons such as fear or misunderstanding, so that they describe only a small proportion of what they feel. This has been called the iceberg phenomenon. Among the troubles often not mentioned are urinary disorders, foot problems, depression and intellectual failure.

Hence old people begin to lose normal functions due to a combination of factors, and doctors now have to learn special skills to be able to assess all the signs and symptoms, and judge the contribution of each. Doctors who specialize in these skills are called geriatricians. Let us consider what they call the four giants of geriatric medicine, the disabling factors that threaten all old people to some degree:

Instability

Immobility

Incontinence

Intellectual failure.

The last is an immense and independent subject that requires a separate chapter of its own.

Instability

What are the causes?

At all ages women are less able than men to maintain an upright posture, but with advancing age it becomes increasingly difficult for both sexes and this in itself causes instability while walking. We have to distinguish though between decline in postural control and falls due to physical disorders. Apart from physical disability, a slowing up of the brain processes which perceive and integrate the messages arriving from the muscles and joints, and the other psychological aspects, play a large part. Some old people become indifferent to danger, while others are accident prone because of impatient and irritable behaviour, from tiredness and emotional upsets.

Almost all old people suffer from dizziness at one time or another. Often it is due to disturbances of the organs of balance and their nervous connections, or to disturbances of the circulation (see also Chapter 3). Another frequent cause of instability is what is called postural hypotension, a feeling of faintness when rising from a sitting position or getting up from a lying down position. This occurs because an older person's blood vessels leading to the brain have hardened, and moving into the upright position causes a temporary reduction in the amount of blood reaching the brain. It may also happen if your relative is taking drugs to lower blood pressure. Such episodes are quite unnerving, and for this reason it is best to have your relative examined by the doctor after a bout of instability. In most cases all that is needed is advice on rising slowly (see below) and reassurance.

More seriously, there are varying degrees of instability caused by arthritis and stroke. For these, advice on rehabilitation from the doctor or physiotherapist will be needed.

While about half the causes of falling are due to the individual's instability, the other half are avoidable hazards in the environment, such as slippery floors, poor lighting and awkward stairs (see also page 22).

Preventing falls

Dizziness on getting up from bed or a chair can be prevented simply by moving more slowly, or getting up in two stages, first to the sitting position, then standing after a short interval for adjustment. Dizziness on rising is particularly common at night, when there is a significant drop in blood pressure. The warmth of the bed increases the bloodflow in the skin so that the brain is relatively starved. Providing a commode or bedpan near the bed, or for men, a urine bottle and a bedside light, are sensible safeguards.

Whenever possible it is preferable for old people to avoid using two canes, so adopting a forward leaning position, and be encouraged to walk upright with just one. However, for people with specific stability problems (for example, anyone with arthritis or who has had a stroke), the tripod and quadropod walking aids are particularly useful. They are made of lightweight aluminium and are of adjustable height, with strong rubber grips on the base. Where even more support is needed two canes are better than the cumbersome pulpit walking frame.

If your relative is living alone you must ensure that he or she will know how to get up after a fall. The illustrations opposite demonstrate the best way, using the stronger arm first, then the stronger foot. When this is not possible your relative must be able to summon help. Much of the anxiety about falling will be removed with the knowledge that help is near by. There are various ways of arranging this, such as having a cane close by to knock on an adjoining neighbour's wall or installing a special alarm system for summoning help after a fall. One is worn on the wrist like a watch and is linked by telephone to an agency who will call up the old person's relatives. Another system is a wire fitted around the

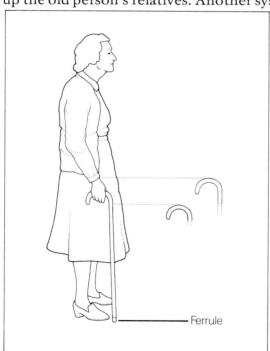

Ferrule

A walking stick should come to the crease in the wrist. If it is too short the elderly person leans forward too much, if too long the stick does not give any support but has to be carried!

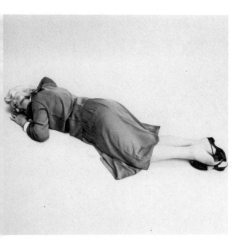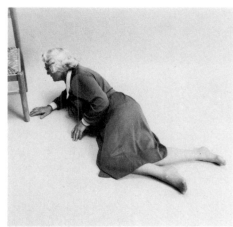

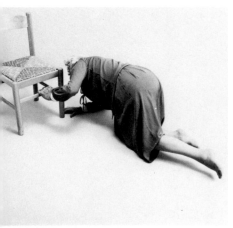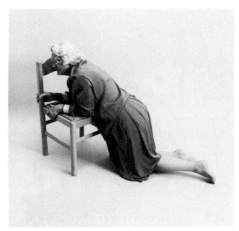

Rising after a fall alone: move on to your stronger side and if possible position yourself near some support. Begin to rise, first using the stronger arm to bear your weight, then the leg. Once on your knees use the support to balance you.

edge of the room which when pulled lights up a sign in the window for help. These are costly and, in the latter case, unless your relative is able to move after falling, they are of no use; hence instability is a serious consideration when deciding on whether someone can live alone safely (see Chapter 2).

The dangers of falling

The majority of falls produce no injury, but breaking bones due to osteoporosis is a major problem for older people, particularly women who are vulnerable after the menopause, since they can become deficient in calcium due to hormonal changes. For this reason it is helpful to increase the daily intake of calcium (see Chapter 3).

Hypothermia Old people who cannot get up after a fall, even though they have no fracture, are in danger of developing hypothermia after lying for a long period on the floor. This is a very real risk among old people living alone. It can develop unnoticed by visiting relatives, and during cold winters is a major cause of death. Falling and being unable to get up is one way that an old person can get hypothermia. Another reason may be an unspoken worry about money – if your relative is frightened of not being able to pay bills, he or she may be cutting down on heating, warm clothing and food.

The condition of hypothermia is described as the point when the deep body temperature, that is, the internal temperature, falls below 95°F (35°C). At this stage the old person will be becoming unconscious and need hospital treatment. But how do you recognize the signs and prevent this happening in the first place?

- During cold weather make frequent calls
- Watch for signs of quietness and withdrawal
- A cold room
- Your relative's skin feeling cold to the touch
- Inadequate clothing.

Often older people living alone have become accustomed to and do not notice the coldness of their environment; sometimes they resent being 'interfered with'. You will have to be tactful in trying to discover the true nature of the problem, and equally tactful in suggesting solutions. Some useful steps to reduce the risks of hypothermia are:

1. Install an easily visible thermometer with the minimum low temperature for the room clearly marked. Some are on sale that have the whole low temperature area coloured blue, so the danger point is easily recognized by an old person. If they are not available in your area, you could mark a large size thermometer yourself.

At all costs, tell your relative not to let the room temperature fall below the low point (65°F or 18°C). Insulating doorways and window frames makes a significant difference in maintaining room temperature and reducing heating bills.

2. Make sure your relative wears plenty of clothes, even in bed; nighttime is especially dangerous with temperatures falling to their lowest, so it is sensible to wear gloves, a cap and several sweaters in very cold weather.

3. Encourage your relative not to stay indoors all day. This cuts people off from social life and leads to further withdrawal and inactivity.

4. See that your relative is eating enough to provide the body with fuel against the cold.

Immobility

Every endeavour should be made to fight immobility. Once your relative is inactive serious complications are likely to develop; besides, the physical and mental strains placed on you are far greater. Although this danger is becoming well-known, it is surprising how many people still retire to bed the moment they feel ill.

But taking up an invalid existence is not the only way of becoming immobile. There is naturally a tendency to slow down with advancing age, and these conditions of aging are contributors:

Obesity
Painful feet
Breathlessness
Arthritis
Visual problems
Stroke
Parkinson's disease.

Obesity

There is always a gain in body fat in women of advancing age, and in a large proportion of men. Even thin old people carry more fat than they did in their youth.

Fatness is rarely the cause of immobility, but is always a strong contributing factor. The obese are also prone to many other diseases. For the overweight elderly person, losing weight is a difficult and in many cases an impossible task. Of course, the same principles of at least preventing excessive weight gain always apply – by eating less fat and sugar, and more fibre, while increasing the energy expenditure.

Any form of exercise is beneficial if it is enjoyed without a sense of strain. Few people will come to any harm if they increase the amount of exercise they take gradually. Walking an extra mile (1.5 km) a day can reduce an elderly person's weight by about 2 lb (1 kg) a month. See Chapter 3 for more advice on appropriate exercise for your relative.

Painful feet

Some years ago I saw a lady of ninety-four who had not been out for six years, and eventually I realized that she had painful, deformed feet. Having her fitted with a specially made pair of surgical shoes worked wonders, and she was able to walk around again. She lived to be a hundred.

Foot complaints are often associated with arthritis, and then medical treatment has to be given. They are also, though, frequently caused by lack of simple care. Skin conditions, nails penetrating the tissues and walking difficulties could often have been prevented. I have emphasized the importance of walking to preserve health, mobility and independence. Looking after your relative's feet is a simple routine that will pay dividends. For practical advice on avoiding painful feet, see Chapter 3.

Breathlessness

This is another contributing factor that has already been touched upon. The effect on mobility is a vicious circle: breathlessness, whether caused by illness or lack of fitness, discourages physical effort so that all movement becomes increasingly difficult.

It is often not easy to know whether old people's breathlessness is due to aging or not. The illnesses causing breathlessness are usually heart disease or chronic lung disease. Other reasons for it may be the effects of drugs, anaemia or emotional disturbance. A lack of fitness is undoubtedly often the reason for breathlessness.

How do you decide the cause if your relative has difficulty breathing? A sudden reduction of capacity to breathe when exercising is likely to be due to illness. Continual breathlessness or difficulty after minimal effort is also a cause for concern. In these cases you should consult the doctor (see also Chapter 3).

Visual problems

I have already described the common conditions that affect elderly people's sight. Whatever the cause, visual failure becomes a great emotional problem which can produce anxiety and depression, and a serious threat to mobility. In Chapter 3 I gave advice on making the best of reduced or restricted vision. A mild form of cataract or macular degeneration will not seriously hamper mobility.

A small proportion of old people do become totally blind. Yet many registered as blind retain enough vision to move around the house. An old person should be encouraged to use all remaining visual power to the full, and not to give up. Looking after a blind person requires some specialized skills. For instance, you have to know how much and what type of guidance is needed, remember to give warning when someone is approaching and provide aids for mobility and communication in the home. Much help can be obtained from agencies for the blind, and public libraries often have information available.

Arthritis

Arthritic pain is extremely common in old age. As many as 10 per cent of the population suffer from the many types of arthritis, and this proportion increases among the elderly. It is important for the condition to be correctly diagnosed. The commonest form is called osteoarthritis. This is not inflammatory, but produced by the wear and tear on joints, affecting mostly the weight-bearing joints, the knees, spine and the hips. It is natural for anyone with osteoarthritis to try and avoid pain by prolonged sitting, but this has the effect of wasting the muscles in the thighs from disuse. For people with a mild form, I urge exercise, perhaps with medication for pain relief. Advanced cases can now be treated by replacement of certain joints such as the hip or knee joint. The operation is costly and its effect lasts for a limited period so that it is usually delayed until immobility is a serious problem. The contrast in increased mobility after a joint replacement is astonishing.

Rheumatoid arthritis is more common in women than men, but overall affects fewer than osteoarthritis – 3 per cent of the population. Usually, but not always, it starts in the small joints of the hands and feet. Eventually other tissues apart from the joints are affected, so that it is a general disease, and not only an inflammation of the joints like osteoarthritis. The body's autoimmune system breaks down as new antibodies attack the body's antibodies. Treatment may be prolonged but in time the condition can burn itself out, leaving joint deformity of varying degrees.

Anyone with severe arthritis will need the help of a physiotherapist. Not only will he or she help your relative keep the joints mobile, but will demonstrate exercises to build up muscle strength and teach control and coordination of movement for everyday activities. This may involve learning to use apparatus or having special equipment installed, such as handrails, or chairs that are easy to rise from.

What can you do to help relieve this painful condition? Above all, encourage your relative to follow the doctor's and physiotherapist's advice:

- If drugs are part of the treatment, make sure they are taken at the

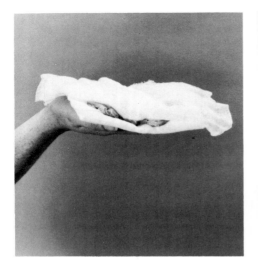
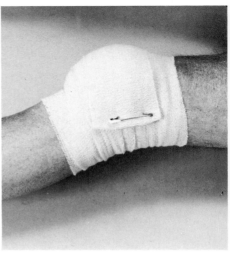

For a painful arthritic knee, a warm poultice can help. Spread heated kaolin on lint and cover with gauze to protect the knee. Make sure the poultice is not too hot. *Right*, place gauze-side down on the knee and secure with firm, not tight bandage.

right times, and watch out for developing side effects.

- See that gentle exercise is taken regularly, according to instructions
- When joints are especially painful and inflamed you can apply either a warm or cold compress, whichever seems to give the most relief
- Suggest your relative has a warm bath on rising in the morning; this will help stiffness after hours of lying in bed
- It may be worth trying acupuncture or seeing an osteopath or chiropracter to relieve pain; these forms of alternative medicine are a great help to many people. You must choose a reputable specialist with the proper qualifications.

The effort to prevent the chairbound or bedridden state is never too great. (See also *Overcoming Arthritis* by Dr Frank Dudley Hart, in this series.)

Stroke

This is a major factor, often causing permanent disability. Because of increasing numbers of stroke cases among older people, many are not admitted to the hospital (in the UK 1 in 250 people over sixty-five has a stroke). It is important for relatives to understand the causes of stroke, and how to look after a patient at home.

Stroke occurs where there is an interruption of the blood supply to the brain. This is due to a vein leading to the brain becoming blocked or an artery bleeding into the brain, or a clot of blood (an embolism) causing a blockage. Before a stroke, there are often warning symptoms such as temporary loss of speech, or function in a limb. These are known as transient ischaemic attacks (TIAs), caused by intermittent blocking in the arteries, and they may allow the doctor to prevent or reduce the severity of stroke.

What are the symptoms?   How do you know that your relative is having a stroke? The exact effect depends on the part of the brain and the amount of brain tissue that is damaged. The brain has four areas controlling different functions – movement, feeling, seeing and hearing (see page 84). It is also divided into two hemispheres, each controlling the opposite side of the body, so that movement is controlled by the left side of the brain in right-handed people, and by the right side in left-handed people. Symptoms of stroke are:

- Loss of speech
- Paralysis
- Loss of feeling in an arm or leg
- Abnormal social behaviour
- Visual disturbance.

One or several of these functions may be impaired. It is common for feeling or movement in one side of the body to be lost (known as hemiplegia), when one hemisphere of the brain is affected. Right-handed people who have a right-sided stroke usually also have their speech affected.

In many ways, the two hemispheres have different functions, so that although it may not seem so bad to have a left-sided stroke, the important function of being able to orient yourself within a confined area is affected. Serious emotional and psychological effects can also result, so that the personality may be greatly altered. It is easier to cope once you realize this is part of your relative's illness rather than anger or depression caused by minor disagreements.

Home care after a stroke
It must be remembered that a stroke's effect is greatest at the time it occurs, and there is often a degree of spontaneous improvement. The chances of recovery are of course affected by the person's age and state of health before the stroke. Older people are far less likely to die from a

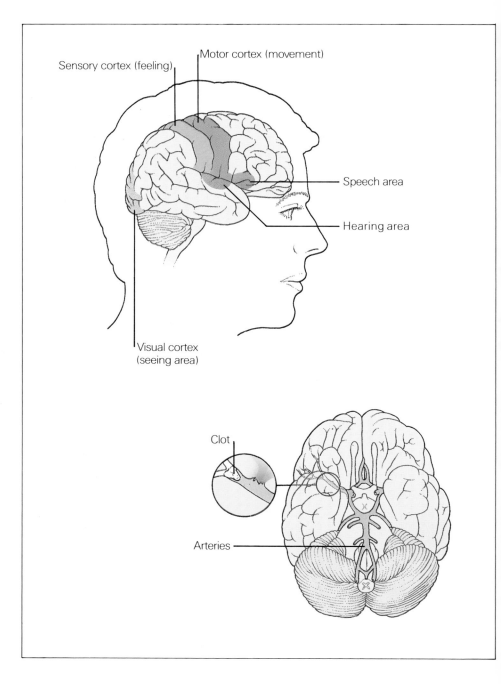

Above The areas of the brain governing different functions. *Below* A stroke may be caused by a clot (embolism) or a haemorrhage in the brain.

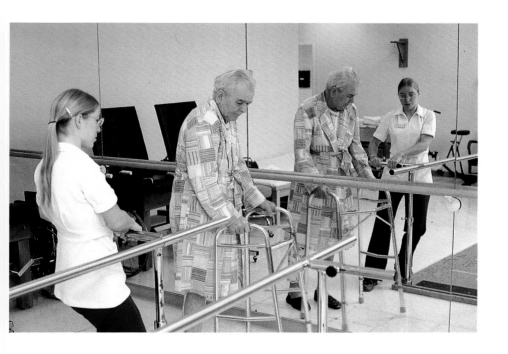

After a stroke that has made mobility difficult, the physiotherapist will teach the correct way to walk.

stroke than middle-aged people. After a few days there will be a noticeable improvement in your relative's condition. Your doctor will suggest the appropriate treatment.

It is very important to begin rehabilitation as soon as some movement is possible. Even a couple of days kept motionless in bed may be harmful, leading to permanent stiffness. You will be shown appropriate exercises by a physiotherapist to help prevent stiffness of muscles and deformity of joints, and you will have to help by continuing them until the muscle spasms are significantly reduced.

Speech therapy may also be needed. The inability to speak is a very complex business, involving a specific impairment of part of the brain. Expert diagnosis of what your relative understands and perceives is necessary before any improvement in speaking can be taught.

When recovery is advanced after some months, it may be especially encouraging for your relative to get out and meet others who are in a similar situation. In many areas now stroke clubs have been started where continuing therapy and social contact have proved a great success. If there isn't a stroke club in your district, why not start one yourself?

Parkinson's disease

This is another disease affecting mobility, especially in elderly people. Although it may start in younger people it is much more common in the old. As many as 1 person in 100 over sixty-five has it in some degree.

Most people can recognize the fully blown picture, but in the early stages it often goes unnoticed. There are three main symptoms:

- Tremor, which may affect one or both hands, or the head; it leads to embarrassment, and clumsiness
- Stiffness of muscles, leading to an expressionless face, stooping and a characteristic way of moving
- A general slowing of movement.

Because the features of this disease are so similar to normal age changes, it is often not until a dramatic event happens, like a fall, that you or the doctor may think something is wrong.

If your relative seems to have aged rather quickly and become forgetful, complains of pains in the neck or shoulders, or is especially depressed; if his or her face seems to have grown expressionless and childlike, you may suspect the early stages of Parkinson's disease. As this is a difficult diagnosis, you will have to ask the doctor to make the necessary detailed examination.

Home care

Luckily, drugs have been discovered that will control Parkinson's disease effectively. Even when these are prescribed, though, your relative will need help. You will have to make many allowances for difficulty in getting around:

- It takes a long time to eat, so keep the food warm by investing in a plate warmer (there are both electric platewarmers and those heated by small candles for sale).
- Keep meals small but with concentrated nutritional value, as slow chewing can make adequate nourishment a problem. As well as sufficient protein, make sure there is enough fibre in the meals, to reduce the possibility of constipation.
- It is unlikely that physiotherapy will be needed, but you should encourage regular walking and muscle stretching; you can mark the floor in an effort to lengthen your relative's paces to 20 in (50 cm).
- There are a number of simple, practical aids to mobility that should not be overlooked:
  – providing heel-less shoes

– and thick handled felt-tipped pens, or even a typewriter for writing
– making sure flooring is even
– setting up a daytime area where all your relative's needs are close by: books, table, lamp, telephone and toilet
– raising the bed on blocks so that it is easier to get into and out of.

Incontinence

Normal control over passing urine is so fundamental to most of us that we don't ever think about it. Yet this demands a series of basic skills involving:

1. Starting at a suitable time, being able to postpone when necessary and to anticipate the need to urinate well in advance
2. Starting to pass water as a voluntary act when the bladder is partly full, being able to control and interrupt if necessary
3. Postponing bladder emptying during sleep and responding by waking in time when the bladder is full
4. Identifying the places or circumstances where it is socially acceptable to pass water, and being able to use the facilities provided.

What we usually take for granted is, after all, quite complicated! Failure is not something people freely discuss, and the symptoms may be concealed for various reasons – shame, or fear that incontinence may force them into institutional care.

What are the causes?
When you realize your relative has this difficulty, it is important to detect the reason, to know if it is a reversible condition or not. Your family doctor may be able to do this, otherwise he or she may call for special tests.

Put simply, the cause is either specific to one part of the body – such as enlarged prostate, prolapse of the womb or stretching caused by childbirth, constipation, or bladder stones, an infection, or the result of certain drugs; in these cases the problem will be solved after successful medical treatment; or it is due to more generalized failure of nervous transmission, such as may happen after a stroke, spinal injury, or some forms of brain disorder.

Finally, don't forget your relative may not be incontinent because of a particular condition. The urge to pass water pretty frequently and quickly is a fact of later life when muscle control is not so good as it used to be.

So long as you make the right provision for someone who is incontinent at home, you should avoid a lot of discomfort and embarrassment. In Chapter 2 we discussed important features of planning the bedroom and bathroom area. Here are some additional points you should consider in relation to incontinence.

Coping with incontinence

1. Is your relative's room more than fifteen paces from the toilet?

2. Could the height or position of the bed or chair be improved?

3. Is he or she taking drugs, such as diuretics, that encourage passing water?

4. Is there good lighting, constant hot water and all around warmth in winter?

5. If your relative is incontinent and confined to bed, how often is he or she changed, and does he spend all the time in night clothes?

When looking after someone who is bedridden, it is particularly important to check for incontinence. Nothing could be more demoralizing and humiliating than being left unchanged.

For someone with permanent difficulty, there are many aids that your family doctor can advise you about, for example, methods of toilet training, and special clothing such as dresses that open at the back. Do not reduce the amount of fluid your relative has in an effort to avert incontinence. This may cause worse problems of dehydration and even confusion.

Faecal incontinence

This is less common than urinary incontinence, but it is equally, if not more, distressing for both you and your relative. Usually the cause is neurological, that is, there is an interruption of the normal mechanisms that control evacuation, due maybe to a stroke or Parkinson's disease. And in many cases, the brain itself fails to register the need in the mind of the old person. We mentioned in Chapter 3 the loaded rectum as a cause of spurious diarrhoea, and this may be another reason for soiling.

At all costs, avoid treating your relative like a naughty child, or with disgust. Try to understand, and this will bring a feeling of sympathy instead of hostility.

There are various ways of making the situation tolerable. Reminding about and encouraging regular habits is the first step. This is not easy, though, and a regular enema to clear the system will make incontinence between evacuations less likely. Your doctor may recommend certain drugs to reduce excessive intestinal activity.

With the three major physical disabilities of old age comes the need for constant and increasing awareness on your part. The fourth disability, intellectual failure, presents further challenges to the carer as it progresses randomly and often with distressing effects on an old person's behaviour. In the next chapter we try to clarify what is happening and suggest how to make things easier for both you and your relative.

6 INTELLECTUAL FAILURE

Loss of competence is frequently but incorrectly attributed to getting old. Very often, what we think to be decline in an old person's mental powers is the result of emotional problems, such as depression or anxiety, or simply disuse; young people kept in solitary confinement need retraining to regain mental competence. Often we overcompensate for old people's mental decline:

A colleague working at Harvard University began to suspect that, however well-meaning, the very act of helping old people may reduce their ability to look after themselves. The opportunities for practising a necessary skill are removed, and the message that they are becoming incapable of self-care, producing a state called 'learned helplessness', is subtly conveyed.

Three groups of old people were given jigsaw puzzles to test their performance. An examiner sat in on one group, encouraging, suggesting where to put pieces, and actively assisting in finding pieces to fit. In another, the examiner gave only minimal assistance and encouragement. In the third group there was no examiner, except for assessment before and after the experiment.

The people who were helped performed less well than those who were only encouraged, while they did less well than those who were left to themselves. The 'helped' group completed on the average fewer pieces, and worked more slowly.

This suggests that, although helpers mean well, they may be reducing the competence of older people in their charge. It also shows that being helped may make a task seem more difficult than it is and so reduce self-confidence.

This does not mean, of course, that the many frail, aged people who require assistance for their very survival should have it withdrawn! But we must judge carefully when to interfere. The old idea that you were always losing brain cells over the age of sixty seemed bad enough, but now we learn that the big losses are when we are younger. In fact the present theory is that we are born with brain cells in excess of normal requirements and are losing a daily quantity from birth. The greatest loss is around the age of forty when we begin to notice failing memory. However, from the start we have learned to do without the ones that become discarded. Mental skills requiring most flexibility are lost quite early – children and young teenagers take to computers and solve the Rubik cube better than anyone. But our ability to make judgments on the basis of information already acquired continues to develop throughout life.

We must therefore make certain whether or not an old person's mental failure is intellectual, and this may require testing by someone specially trained. We are all familiar with remarkable people who preserve their mental powers and personality intact into the nineties. We are also painfully aware that many become depressed and lose their mental acuity. For the majority there is a falling off in certain mental abilities, particularly those tasks that require a solution within a given time. There is a slowing of response due to delay within the central nervous system, and so patience is needed in communication, and instructions are best given simply and briefly to allow plenty of time for absorption. Old people find doing two things at once difficult, so you may see an old lady stop walking while she puts on her gloves. Then again you may notice old people moving their lips while reading, and this is because they need to reinforce their understanding by hearing the words as well as seeing them.

Of course it is characteristic for the elderly to become less adaptable, as we already discussed in Chapter 2, and this can make them difficult to live with. Even more important, perhaps, it may be a serious barrier to successful rehabilitation after an illness when new skills have to be learned. In this chapter we describe the different ways your relative's mental processes may be affected and how you may have to cope with these problems of the mind.

Normal changes of aging

The emotions   In old people, emotions assume an increasingly dominant role and are liable to colour their beliefs about their lifestyle. There may be a blunting of feeling leading to apathy or indifference, or an accentuation of former characteristics so that someone, say, who used to be strict and have demanding standards either mellows into tolerance or hardens into despotism. It is well known that emotional activity in the elderly tends towards certain patterns of behaviour – resistance to change, lack of spontaneity, greater caution and distrust of the unfamiliar.

Memory   It is often said that when you are old you can remember the distant past, but not what has just happened. This distinction, however, is not by any means clear-cut. We have a short-term memory and a faculty for retaining information, such as shopping lists, for a short time only, and then discarding it when it is no longer needed. Certainly

8.00	Wash and dress	3.30	
8.30	Exercise routine	4.00	Tea break
9.00	Breakfast	4.30	
9.30		5.00	Watch television
10.00	Day Club (fake basketwork)	5.30	
10.30		6.00	
11.00	Coffee break	6.30	
11.30		7.00	
12.00		7.30	Evening meal
12.30	Midday meal	8.00	
1.00		8.30	Help with washing up
1.30		9.00	
2.00	Bus from Club home	9.30	
2.30		10.00	Bedtime drink
3.00	Rest and read.	10.30	Bed.

An example of a daily diary – for a very forgetful relative more detail can be added for each activity.

when someone's brain starts to fail, short-term memory is more vulnerable, but this is really because of an inability to register the information in the first place.

We all begin to notice that our memory is not so good once we have passed forty, and this type of forgetfulness is characterized by difficulty in recalling names and events. Loss of recent memory – or indeed of any period involving whole episodes, is a different type of failure and should be regarded as a symptom of disease rather than a feature of aging. This may be due to a number of conditions, both physical and mental (stroke or alcoholism, or dementia, see page 94), and including the effect of drugs. So a good medical opinion based on experienced assessment is needed.

Memory aids   There are many practical ways you can suggest to help your relative remember necessary facts and domestic details. These will both provide confidence and can act as a form of memory training:

1. Keep a large daily diary with space to write all the day's activities, hour by hour

2. Use details in the environment – definite times, places, objects – to act as reminders to do a particular task. For example, put the coffee jar in a prominent place in the kitchen so that preparing a routine mid-morning snack is remembered

3. Reduce daily activities to those that are easily remembered by your relative

4. Encourage occupations that do not tax the memory too much, for example, painting or gardening

5. Praise, even reward good recall, but avoid putting your relative to the test.

Quite often elderly people lose their sense of identity, and need to be reminded who they are, where they are and what time of day it is. Keeping clocks and calendars, family pictures and mementos on hand so that your relative can refer to them constantly helps strengthen self-confidence. Make sure these aids are large, clearly marked and accurate. Reminiscence can be used as a pleasurable form of mental stimulation. But when old people begin to ramble, it is a good idea to change the subject to something more concrete. Encourage your relative to make choices, and so retain his or her independence.

These suggestions are useful for everyone with a degree of memory failure. They can also be helpful in stimulating elderly people with more severe mental disability.

Mental disorder

The idea of mental failure   I want to say that whereas medical labels are useful to the profession, I am not speaking only of dementia here. True dementia is irreversible, but the brain may fail – that is, become confused – for many other reasons, which are reversible. We have to think of mental failure rather in the same way as we do cardiac failure. This means that it can be compensated for and kept going with various forms of help, such as I suggest above. The necessary adjustment can be made by reducing incoming strains and providing a simple, familiar routine. Perhaps the most important task for the doctor is to distinguish the elements of dementia and confusion from treatable depression, and this is not easy.

Confusion

Confusion can unfortunately give a false impression of dementia. But it is simply a descriptive term indicating that someone has a disordered awareness of his or her surroundings. Of course you can be confused more easily when you are dementing – but anyone submitted to too many stimuli can be made confused. Old people who cannot discriminate between sights and sounds are predisposed, so that confusion is particularly common at dusk, when it is difficult to pick things out from the background and stereoscopic (simultaneous) vision is much reduced.

A state of confusion may be accompanied by delusions. Perhaps you have felt confused for a moment on waking up in a strange hotel, or when suddenly questioned while daydreaming? On a lazy holiday you may not be able to say what day or time of day it is. So remember that anyone can become confused in situations where too much or too little is happening, the surroundings are unfamiliar and emotional drives are strong.

In fact, if your relative is only confused, you can feel optimistic about the outcome. In many cases confusion can be treated by removing the cause, which may be one or a combination of the following:

- A full bladder
- Constipation
- The effect of drugs
- An infection
- Heart disease
- Minor stroke.

Looking after a confused person requires skilful handling. It is important not to thwart, but to learn how to guide and soothe your relative. If, for instance, your old father has got up in the night with the idea of going to work it is better to say, 'Can I come along too?' and lead him into the kitchen to sit down and wait for the bus, than to get into a noisy confrontation. After a while he may take a glass of milk or a hot drink and quietly return to bed, having forgotten where he was going in the first instance. Let me say at once that this cannot always work, but it is the approach most likely to succeed.

Dementia

Although it is so prevalent in old age – it has been estimated that about one person in five over the age of eighty suffers from moderate or severe dementia – it is not easy to detect at first. If you notice that your relative has serious memory lapses, as I explained on page 92, or starts to behave in unusual or obsessional ways, or has trouble with language, you should speak to your doctor about it. Any of these may be due to anxiety or drug effects, to confusion, or to brain damage, so skilled testing will be needed to decide what is at the root.

Coping with dementia At least eight in ten elderly people with dementia are cared for at home and they are also likely to be affected with other mental and physical illness, imposing a severe strain on the relatives caring for them. Depending on the degree of dementia, there will be repetition, restlessness, mistaking people's identity – even yours – lack of motivation, memory lapses, hitting out at supporters, and disturbances at night. Falls and incontinence are caused by lack of physical control and the sufferer's unawareness of his or her own body.

I think it is true to say that the wish to care for someone with these problems grows out of an established pattern of life, reinforced by bonds of affection and obligation. But, of course, the personality change and the accompanying problems mean you will feel sadness, and at times exasperation, more acutely. When you care for someone in this condition, one of the worst features is the inability to sustain a conversation. It seems as if the person is gradually becoming more and more remote, although the physical resemblance is there.

What should you look out for if you suspect your relative has dementia? The following are typical symptoms; they can be alleviated provided you are alert to them and take the measures suggested here and by your doctor or geriatrician:

- Poor communication
- Memory loss
- Non-recognition of people
- Over-dependence
- Decreased participation in family life and leisure activities
- Difficulty in maintaining appropriate social behaviour and hygiene.

The problems of confusion and dementia become your responsibility, and that of the rest of the family, so:

DO
- Recognize aspects of the basic personality, hopes and expectations of your relative which are still intact
- Treat him or her as an adult, with dignity – not as a child
- Expect your relative to fulfil responsibilities as a member of the household
- Respond to confusion and disorientation with facts
- Reward accomplishment

DON'T
- Become overprotective, doing everything for your relative
- Focus on lost capacities and overlook those that remain
- Go along with delusions and reinforce them: equally, do not

95

oppose them to the extent of creating anxiety and hostility
- Give in to unreasonable demands

- Reward disability by being over-sympathetic.

The supporter's needs in caring for dementia and confusion

1. Early involvement of services
The strain of caring wears the supporters down, and outside help can prevent or at least reduce this process. Don't wait until you are already exhausted.

You will need to find out what help is available locally and how to go about getting it (see Chapter 9 for agencies you can approach), and what benefits you may be eligible for.

2. Assessment
This should cover all the main problems you and your relative are going to face. You need professional assessment by someone who shows sensitivity, will listen, give you clear explanations, understand the likely causes of confusion in your relative's case, and who can suggest an easily implemented plan of action. In the UK and Australia this is likely to be done by your own doctor. In North America a geriatrician will assess your relative.

You should ask for further assessment by a specialist when intervention is going to be effective, rather than when you feel you have already reached breaking point.

3. Continuing support
The continuing involvement of professionals who are interested, can be called on at difficult times and who will review the situation at regular intervals, is essential.

4. Regular help with household and personal care
You must arrange help in the home with domestic work, if possible, and with laundry – anything that reduces the workload.

5. Skilled medical and nursing treatment
This may be needed during acute episodes, possibly night and day.

6. Regular breaks
Day care and short-term admission to the hospital provides relief for you and maybe stimulation along with the changed environment for your relative. This needs to be planned ahead. Some geriatric depart-

ments organize a rota system with several elderly people alternating, taking turns occupying the same hospital bed for a week at a time. Day care in local centres is also provided in many places, and is very successful for the vast majority. Group occupational therapy re-establishes social links, and maybe a morale boosting hairdo relieves tedium and depression. If there is no such centre in your area, you might consider starting one up as a self-help project.

7. Regular financial support
Ask your doctor or geriatrician whether there is any financial provision for the added expenses incurred by caring for someone with dementia.

8. Permanent residential care
Despite the trend towards care at home or in the community, permanent residential care will continue for those whose relatives cease to be able to look after them, either because of the elderly person's worsening condition or their own inability to cope. Regular assessment ensures that this is arranged when and if it is needed.

Depression

Of the mental disorders, depression is second only to dementia, and in some ways could be said to be more important, for although it causes more suffering it may be treated successfully. Diagnosis of true depression is not always easy (see also Chapter 3). I suppose there is a psychology of every age, and old people become slower and less optimistic than the young. But this does not mean they have a condition requiring medical treatment.

Nevertheless, any depression has a very pervasive effect. Old people who are depressed may be thought to have dementia because they cannot remember and concentrate as they should, and are generally slower in thinking. But there are differences in the symptoms:

- There is a loss of interest and drive, appetite and weight, and an exaggerated appearance of aging
- Sleep is interrupted, particularly in the early morning hours
- Sometimes the sufferer is agitated and restless
- Expressions of emptiness, hopelessness, dissatisfaction and demoralization are the clearest indications of a depression
- Eventually delusions, especially about bowel function, and even suicidal thinking, are possible.

You should seek your doctor's advice if your relative is very depressed. Early treatment is important. Should the condition become chronic, a long period of rehabilitation will be necessary. The normal treatment is with drugs. These are not without side effects, and they take perhaps a month to raise the mood, but they quickly improve appetite and the quality of sleep.

The drugs, which have a twenty-four hour action, are often given all at once, early in the evening. Taken at this time, the maximal effect is when early waking and rumination usually begin. After they have relieved the depression, your relative may be able to do without them; otherwise a low maintenance dosage will be advised.

Paranoia of old age

Strangely enough, there are sex differences in mental illness, and in the elderly this one occurs almost exclusively amongst aged women! Whereas a depressed old person blames his or her painful sense of guilt and inadequacy upon himself, and feels he deserves to be punished, the paranoid reaction is at the opposite extreme. Elderly ladies with this condition place all blame on others, whom they regard with increasing mistrust and hostility, and they are constantly at the centre of fruitless and exasperated argument. As with dementia, it is important not to oppose their ideas.

> I remember being called to a country hotel to see an old lady who insisted that some young men were deliberately annoying her by making a noise beneath her window with their motor cycles. The manager had told her son that if she did not stop making complaints she would have to leave. Seven doctors had already seen her, and each one had looked out and reported there were no young men there, so the distressed son told me. Each one had left, making the old lady more anxious as she believed them to be agents of persecution.
>
> I decided a new attitude was needed. When she told me about the noise I said, 'This must be very distressing for you.' She then allowed me to examine her, and I found she had severe cardiac failure which was depriving her brain cells of nutrition. We agreed on a plan of treatment.
>
> A week later, she no longer had heart failure and she was mentally improved. But had her delusions gone? I asked about the nasty young men, and she replied, 'Oh them! Last Monday they drove away, and they haven't returned, thank goodness.'

It is always best to let your relative express her annoyance, and if you can't find a reasonable explanation, ask your doctor to make a sympathetic examination. Don't rule out the possibility of a physical condition causing the paranoia. But if it turns out to be a mental failure, it can be treated with drugs. Encourage as normal a life as possible. Having plenty of social contact, especially with elderly people who are well-disposed, is a great help to a confused and unhappy old lady.

Your role

Distressing though the features of mental failure are, the best care is undoubtedly for close relatives to look after the sufferer at home. They have the advantage over others of having known the elderly person before he or she became ill. You know best whether she was introverted or extroverted, and what principles are held dear. You have shared family stories and common memories, and with these you, more than anyone, can stimulate the interest and emotions. Set time aside for conversation to strengthen the grip on reality: your aim is to retain your relative's personality for as long as possible.

It would be rare for anyone to fulfil the functions discussed, not only in this chapter, but throughout the book, singlehanded and without fatigue. The build up of strain in the carer must be foreseen and avoided. In Chapter 7 I show how looking after yourself and your needs, rather than being selfish, is absolutely necessary if you are to continue to be a help to your relative and to preserve an independent existence for yourself.

7 CARING FOR THE CARER

Real caring is giving, and this involves sacrifice. You are not just a machine, neither is caring a work-like routine. I have seen many cases where this sacrifice has been too great for the carer, so that we professionals have had to be involved in looking after both.

It is not selfish when undertaking a long and heavy task to consider your own health, even to the point of having it assessed by your doctor. It is prudent. It stands to reason that if you are going to care for someone else, you must be healthy yourself. In addition, not only must you start the job of caring in good health, but you must maintain it through every day. A poor mental approach, painful twinges or chronic fatigue diminish anyone's ability to give. You must therefore look at the present position, and the work involved, and estimate carefully the likelihood of increasing dependency and what this will mean.

The advice in this chapter is especially directed towards the single carer, who has no family support. Without a caring relative watching *your* health, it is easy to forget and let yourself become run down. You have to consider your own interests as well as your elderly relative's.

Self-care

This involves both planning and monitoring. We have to assume that you are in good health to start with. So let us look at some of the obvious ways to preserve and even improve your good health for the future.

Your physical health

Diet I have seen many carers who prepare excellent meals for the invalid but take little care over their own food. This is a great mistake. You should always make time to sit down and eat a meal which is planned to be enjoyed. The best foods are fresh vegetables and fruit, wholegrain breads and lean meat or fish. The important things to remember are including sufficient roughage, ensuring freshness and eating in moderation. You never want a meal to make you feel heavy and drowsy. It is better to eat three small meals throughout the day rather than a large one in the evening.

Exercise You may well point out that doing household chores, getting to a workplace or the shops gives you plenty of exercise. Indeed they do, but you should also plan rhythmic exercise to increase and maintain physical fitness. To be effective, this exercise must be pleasurable. It is designed to increase the heart rate gradually, improving circulation and muscle tone. Furthermore, it relaxes the mind (it is difficult to work on problems if you are jogging). There are many ways of taking exercise – a brisk walk lasting at least forty-five minutes, or swimming, are the best forms, especially if you have not been taking regular exercise up to now. Starting with the more vigorous sports such as tennis or squash, or doing aerobics, can be dangerous. If though you are already fit you may enjoy skipping or jogging. And just about everywhere now there are keep fit classes for all ages and abilities. Make sure you choose a programme suitable for your fitness level.

Finally, don't neglect your own body in your concern for your relative's. Take care of any cuts or scratches that may become infected, and have a good first aid kit at hand in case of accidents in the home.

Backache

I have found that of all the physical complaints among carers, backache is the most common. This would seem to be due to too much lifting – moving an immobile person up the bed, or helping an old father out of his chair. Overlifting and straining do of course occur. But often the backache is psychosomatic. It is a way of telling others that the burden is becoming too great. It is no good for doctors to make an examination, find that movement is normal, and say there is nothing wrong. The backache is a stress signal, it is a warning sign and indicates the need for a break from carrying the burden, often singlehanded.

On the matter of lifting, remember that you should not lift heavy weights with your back bent. If you watch Olympic weight lifters, they use their knees, and keep their back straight, and even hollowed. That is what you should always do. You may need to rethink some of the ways you lift – perhaps lifting your relative from behind, instead of in front, or putting a knee right up on the bed to obtain leverage (see also Chapter 4 for advice on lifting).

Sleep

Most people need about seven or eight hours' sleep at night. You will know your own requirements, and they are important in many ways, both physical and mental. When the emotions are disturbed, one of the first things to be upset is the sleep pattern.

It does not matter if the occasional night's sleep is interrupted or shortened, for it can be made up. But, with the demanding task of caring for someone else, you should make every effort to get regular hours of sleep. Using drugs or alcohol to put you to sleep is not a good idea. Alcohol may work at first, but you will probably waken again feeling restless, or needing to go to the toilet. If you feel you have to break a cycle of sleepless nights a non-prescription sleeping tablet recommended by the pharmacist may be effective, but take one only for two or three nights at a time, not as a habit. When sleep becomes a real problem, it is best by far to discuss it with your doctor.

Mental state

Watch your emotional health. Ask yourself whether you laugh and smile now, and if you feel enthusiastic. Is your sleep pattern being disturbed? Do you get up feeling refreshed in the morning? Do you become irritable easily, or want to get away from it all? Everyone has these feelings for short periods, but if they are lengthening and increasing, your emotional health is deteriorating. You may then ask yourself if your needs are being fulfilled, and whether you are being taken for granted, even abandoned by others. You may not realize what is happening to you at first, but very often a frank talk with an understanding friend to whom you can unburden yourself will reveal the problems.

You should consider whether you are becoming dependent on stimulants or tranquillizers, and I include here caffeine, alcohol and tobacco, overeating, especially sweets, as well as prescribed tranquillizers and sleeping pills. If you are starting to rely on a regular intake of any of these you are not doing well. For one thing, the amount tends to increase, while the effect starts to decline. So be realistic with yourself, particularly if no one else knows what you are taking. You may feel that the tranquillizers are relieving stress, but if you cannot do without them, then the right thing is to look for help and advice.

Stress

How can you define stress? The important thing is to understand that if you feel under stress, then you are. Other people do not know. They may think a situation which you find perfectly acceptable is stressful to you, and tell you so. Whether this is true depends on you. You have to sit back and assess the position yourself.

The effect of stress for a short time is something the body is built to deal with. In fact, a little is essential to keep us alert and in good health. Without daily challenges to stimulate us, we become torpid. Prolonged stress is a different matter. It makes you feel permanently tired. Typical effects are:

- Finding simple daily tasks an effort
- Losing a sense of proportion – small problems seem insurmountable
- Feeling you cannot cope
- Loss of sense of humour
- Sleeping badly.

You adapt to a stressful situation and for a time maintain it, until break-

102

down occurs. During the adaptation various physical changes happen, such as a raising of the blood pressure, and alteration of fat levels in the blood, which contribute towards heart disease.

Avoid stress by watching out for the signs that I have described. You must allow yourself time for proper rest and relaxation away from your duties. Later in this chapter I give more advice on this important need. If you do feel things are on top of you and you can't cope, talk to your doctor or a psychiatrist.

Irritability

You will, of course, get irritable at times. You will then blame yourself. It is not always possible to behave perfectly while caring for others, and it can help you cope if you understand what is happening. I suppose people are most likely to become irritable when caring for an old mother or father with a failing brain, who repeats everything they say, remembers nothing and shows coarsening of behaviour. Although you recognize the face of someone you know, love and respect, and on whom you once depended, the roles have become reversed. You have the feeling that your relative is gradually disappearing, and that you are now in the position of the mother or father. This is a strange situation, and one you may not have expected. It will take time to adjust.

The relationships appears different to outsiders, even including your doctor. Quite often an elderly person behaves much better in front of other people than for you, and that is grievous. The fact is that no one else can really understand this hurtful, sad, angry regret that you feel.

Might I strike my own mother?   Yes, quite clearly you might. In the situation of role reversal, and behaviour disorder, the change wrought in your beloved parent can produce sudden confused emotion in you which overflows into shouting and slapping. It is immediately followed, not by satisfaction, but by deep, humiliating guilt, so great in some cases that the carer can no longer continue, and needs care herself.

I have mentioned this because it is not uncommon, yet people rarely talk about it. Only someone actually in this position knows what it is like. But in my experience, it occurs after a long period of devoted caring, when the stress has been mounting, and the carer is becoming exhausted and at the end of her tether. It can and should be foreseen and prevented by giving proper attention to your own needs.

Preserving a life of your own

The business of caring involves sacrifices, and one of them is a loss of social life. Really good friends will continue to visit and offer help, but I fear that human nature is such that people usually stay away. I would therefore urge you to make every effort to retain contact with other people, perhaps just once a week, not as a self-indulgence, but because it will normalize your feelings and restore a sense of proportion and humour. Do not forget also the danger of losing friendships through neglect. Some regular contact will preserve precious relationships for the time when your task is over.

Your other great need is to have a complete break from caring. This should be planned when you start looking after someone, and not as a desperate effort to keep going by way of escape. Such last minute measures will not refresh you and may cause you anxiety and feelings of guilt. A regular holiday, agreed in advance by everyone concerned will, on the other hand, make your job all the more worthwhile to come back to.

Who will stand in while you are having your rest?
For carers with other family members who can take the elderly person for a short stay, arranging a break is simple. It may not seem as easy if you are a single person. However, many hospitals arrange for temporary admission of elderly patients during the summertime, for periods of a couple of weeks. The success of an arrangement like this can lead on to more regular breaks, such as the six-week-in and six-week-out type of shared care, or spending weekends in the hospital.

Alternatively, some nursing homes make flexible arrangements with relatives. If neither of these options is open, you may be able to arrange for a qualified nurse to live in and look after your relative for a while.

In my experience, it is the unremitting task and the feeling that no one else will take responsibility that destroys the morale of the carer. The situation is quite different when care is shared and breaks can be looked forward to. But you have to consider who will best take on the job while you have your break.

Delegating responsibility
People vary in their ability to delegate. There are those who would not dream of letting anyone else look after their mother, while others do not seem to worry unduly who is taking up the burden. It is important to examine your own feelings, and perhaps, motives. What is essential is to choose someone suitable, who is properly qualified to look after your relative and with the ability to care sympathetically for an old person. Examine the references and experience if the helper is a professional, and maintain formal communication during the break. Ask for a daily written record of all medical treatment, and observations on the state of health.

I hope this chapter has convinced you of the value of looking after your health and your own interests. It may be difficult to arrange a perfectly harmonious and independent life for yourself while caring for your relative. But keeping fit mentally and physically should go a long way towards making things easier. The information about external help in Chapter 9 should encourage you in the knowledge that it is not necessary to shoulder the task alone.

8 DYING AT HOME

As we have shown earlier, with improved medical treatments, the elderly today are less likely to die from diseases such as tuberculosis and typhoid fever that were common earlier this century. Death is usually the combination of long-term weakening through the aging process and a final illness.

Will your relative die at home?   Most old people die from heart disease, stroke or cancer. When death is sudden, due to heart disease or stroke, about half die at home. Those with cancer or a rare disease are more likely to die in the hospital.

At present, fewer old people have to be nursed to the end at home, if the relatives prefer not to, but the increasing accent on home care for the elderly may reverse this trend. Whether you will be able to look after your relative right up until the time he or she dies will depend a lot on your own circumstances. The same considerations of family commitments, physical and financial resources and employment that were important in undertaking caring are all the more relevant when deciding on nursing a failing old person. The final illness may be long and tedious, and what was possible for the forty year old may prove impossible for the seventy-five year old daughter or wife.

A pattern of care is often agreed with most of the illness being spent at home, but when the relatives can no longer cope, the old person is admitted to the hospital for the last week or so. People sometimes suffer feelings of guilt and regret that they could not continue their care to the very end. I feel they cannot and should not blame themselves in any way. Terminal nursing often requires specialized skills which few untrained people easily adapt to.

Dying is natural

Despite the great increase in communication and open discussion of biological matters, we in the West remain a death denying society. More than at any other age, death comes to the very young or the very old. Most people have little contact with it, and are frightened and ignorant of what to do. Children are provided with sexual information as soon as they ask where they came from. Their final destiny is never mentioned: even in their teens they are very much overprotected. Our present attitudes are the reverse of the nineteenth century. Then sexual questions were fended off, while death was a regular element of hymns and prayers. Yet, those who have experience of old people dying are unanimous in their testimony that death is nearly always gentle and peaceful.

Answering questions – should you tell?

This is a very individual decision. But it may be interesting to know how often people can and prefer to accept the truth. In a recent British survey, 13 per cent of terminally ill patients were given a frank explanation of their situation, and were able to discuss it openly with their doctor. The doctors themselves considered that about half their dying patients already had a good idea of their real condition. Inevitably, there are people, usually spouses, who ask the doctor not to tell the dying patient the truth because he or she 'couldn't stand it'. This leads to the awkwardness of deception. The dying person is told, 'You must expect to get worse before you can get better', and so on. Of course this causes tension and false emotions. Above all, it prevents a loving couple or parent and child from saying anything meaningful to each other.

A kind and trusted doctor will not act against relatives' wishes, and will always spend time discussing what seems best from everyone's point of view. He or she would never go up to a dying person with the news that death is in sight. If you place trust in your doctor's professional capacity you will find him a tremendous support at this delicate time. He will wait until questions are asked and will have the skill to answer them according to your relative's degree of understanding and emotional maturity. He knows that it is not death that worries people so much as the pain and suffering of dying. And he will be able to offer much reassurance on that score. Above all, the promise of regular visits, even if no treatment is given, are of the greatest help. To the relatives, the doctor's immense value is in providing all the necessary medical information and counselling.

Nursing a dying relative

Without experience, you may be frightened of not recognizing or being able to act when the time comes. In fact, with the knowledge gathered from earlier caring, and your close relationship, this will be less traumatic than you imagine. The need for practical nursing will be like an antidote to distress. The support of your doctor, friends and relatives should help you through.

When constant nursing, day and night, is necessary, you must arrange for assistance. If you have no immediate family who can offer their help, you may be able to call on other members of the family to live in for the necessary time. Otherwise, you will have to organize professional help (special organizations and addresses appear in Chapter 9).

Form the helpers into a team so that someone is always with your relative, while the others are resting. Reporting to each other is important, and it is a good idea to keep an hourly record.

The first aim is to keep your relative comfortable, peaceful and content. Care and attention to physical needs will make this time easier to bear. The details of home nursing as described in Chapter 4 will act as a guide. Some special aspects of nursing a dying person need mentioning here.

Pain Most people dying at home have a certain amount of pain. But psychological and social features have a great effect on its severity. When my own father came home to die from bladder cancer, he was able to do without the morphine he had been given in the hospital. This was because he felt happier and more secure within his own family. On the other hand, those who have no distractions and are left alone feel pain much more acutely.

When someone is dying, pain can be totally prevented, rather than just relieved. This means that the drug dosage and timing must be specially gauged for the individual and you will be given careful instructions by your doctor if you have to administer the drugs. The most commonly used are of the morphine group. There is of course no question of addiction to drugs in terminal illness. Drug doses do not usually need to be increased but this may be a help if you notice excessive discomfort and restlessness, for instance at night, when pain is usually more severe. Ask your doctor about the possibility of this, and how much you might need to increase the dose. I would stress that we don't wait for pain and then relieve it. We give regular doses to prevent it.

There are now specialized pain control clinics that use nerve block and other procedures for exceptional problems. Your doctor would suggest a consultation only if your relative is suffering greatly.

Bed sores We described the problem of bed sores in Chapter 4. Very old, wasted people are particularly prone to them, and need to be turned every hour. They are caused, not by wet sheets, but pressure on certain parts of the body resulting from immobility. Even with constant care, sores are not always preventable. Try to obtain a ripple mattress as soon as possible, for this at least reduces the inevitability of bed sores developing.

Specialized nursing Alleviating nausea and vomiting, dressing open wounds and treating sinuses are among the skills that require the advice of experienced nurses and doctors. Professional assistance with these duties will give you confidence. It is also comforting for your relative to be nursed by someone assured and quick in giving treatment, who knows how to avoid painful movements.

Psychological support Sometimes people know the situation, yet they may not have come to terms with it, or shared it. Their wish to see someone with whom there is a deep personal relationship may be at the root of the anxiety, as it was in one of my patients. She was beautifully cared for by everyone present, but I realized her need was to see the prodigal son, who had for many years gone his own way. He was telephoned, and after he had visited her she had no more pain. Many other people have spiritual needs, which can best be helped by a minister.

What to do when someone dies

The specific procedures after a death vary, depending on where you live. Here I give guidelines applicable to most places.

First you should contact

1. The family doctor. He or she will need to certify that death has occurred, and issue a death certificate. He will tell you also how to register the death.

2. The nearest relative.

3. The relevant minister.

4. If the organs are to be donated the eyes must be removed within six hours, so the nearest eye hospital should be told; kidneys are not likely to be donated by an elderly person.
   Sometimes the body is to be donated, and the appropriate agency has to be informed.

5. Once death has been certified, the body is put flat, the arms placed across the chest, and the eyes closed. These tasks, and washing the body, are usually performed by the relatives. Some people don't like to touch the body and then a nurse must be asked to do it.

6. In the normal circumstances of a natural death, once the written certificate has been issued by the doctor, the funeral directors can be contacted, who will fulfil the family's further wishes. For instance they will help you to decide:

   ● Where the body will await the funeral
   ● The starting point, time and place of the funeral
   ● Whether there will be a funeral service

- Whether the dead person is to be buried or cremated
- Whether you want flowers, or donations to a named charity.

These steps you have to take immediately. Later you must give attention to the legal aspects:

- The registration of the death
- Whether there is a will, and who the executor is
- If there is no will, letters of administration must be obtained
- What about taxes? You need financial and legal advice
- Did your relative rent or own the home? If so, what are your rights?
- Don't overlook returning passport, driving licence, membership cards, credit cards and so on.

Finally you have to sort out and dispose of your relative's belongings. This is both a chore and a cause of distress. Try and get someone to help you, and don't consider starting until you feel you have the strength – perhaps a few weeks after the funeral.

Was it all worth it?

For most of us the greatest satisfaction in life comes from helping others. There is a sense of fulfilment after a well-directed effort has been made, and the reward has little to do with expressed gratitude, although it gives pleasure.

People who care for a very old and frail relative often find they are looking after someone quite out of touch with what is going on. No outsider can really understand the personal nature of such relationships. Many people have told me that if they had known how things would develop they would not have dared begin, but that during the task they have found added strength they had not imagined possible. At the beginning, most find themselves clumsy, faulty and disorganized, yet it always interests me how quickly people learn new skills, and learn from their mistakes. While some are natural nurses, others need help and encouragement.

I remember a young man and his two married sisters deciding to look after their widowed mother at home. She was dying of cancer. The younger sister, not long married, took to nursing as if she had done it all her life. The other, the mother of two small boys, could not go up to the bedroom. But her seven year old son insisted on seeing his grandmother. He sat on the bed, unaffected by her wasted frame and inability to speak. He just played a game on the bed.

When the four year old wanted to see her too, I was asked if he should. Knowing that children are more realistic than adults, I was less concerned that he should see his grandmother not looking her best than that he should not be made afraid of death. He too visited the old lady and seemed quite unperturbed. After that, the children's mother followed, and was able to help her sister with the nursing.

During my thirty years' experience I have had many people tell me of their now inconsolable regret, and even guilt, that a loved parent spent the end of their lives in a hospital or home, cared for by others. In some cases it has produced years of grim remorse, with profound effect on family and working life. We all have unfinished business with our parents. But I can truthfully say that where the relative has undertaken the care at home this has never been the case.

For the home carer, a further reward comes at the end. The period after death, which we call bereavement, does not follow the usual pattern. The mourning and grieving have been expressed during the period of caring, and the fact of death has simply released each of you, usually with relief on both sides. The carer feels a sense of freedom and achievement, and a permanent exaltation in the relationship that led to the caring at home in the first place. So far as I have been able to judge, these feelings are not affected by drained energy or dwindled finances. It is very much a situation in which you reap what you have sown.

9 WHERE CAN YOU GET HELP?

Support services for the carer vary from one country to another and even from area to area, depending often on funds available. As it is not possible to describe each and every system in detail, in this chapter we describe the overall picture in the different countries relevant to readers, and list the principal organizations where help can be obtained. We have emphasized often throughout the book how important it is to inform yourself at the beginning about all the external aid you might need at any one time. Financial support is always important and you should inquire as soon as you take over responsibility for your relative whether you are entitled to any, and what grants or tax reliefs may be open to you.

United Kingdom

Medical help
The first person to turn to is your family doctor, who will be able to advise you on the minor ailments described in Chapters 3 and 4. Your relative will be referred by the doctor to a geriatrician, and admission to hospital will be organized if needed for investigation and treatment of major illnesses.

If your relative can be nursed at home, the services of a district nurse or a health visitor may be arranged through your doctor. If you are unable to cope with the physical burden – say your relative is immobilized by a minor stroke – you may also ask for a home help to come once or twice a week to assist with bathing and other heavy duties. This service, and others such as meals on wheels, are organized by the local authorities, and the amount available varies according to where you live. You can get information about help from the social services department in your area or from organizations for the elderly.

Chiropody Elderly people are entitled to free chiropody on the National Health Service, though in many areas there are long waiting lists. Your doctor will direct you to the chiropodist providing this service in your area.

Shared care
Day centres These are organized by local authorities, often in con-

junction with the major charities and with voluntary helpers. They are invaluable in keeping elderly people stimulated. Attendance for a day or two each week also relieves the carer of responsibility for that time. They are not to be confused with day hospitals.

Day hospitals   These are provided in all health regions. Medical treatments, bathing, hairdressing, occupational and physiotherapy are given. This avoids the need to stay in hospital. But hospital patients also attend, and the day hospitals are a halfway stage between hospital and the community.

Holidays   The options of admitting an infirm elderly person to the hospital while the carer takes an annual holiday, or arranging a short term stay at a nursing home, are mentioned in Chapter 7. Nursing homes in the UK are either under the local authority or privately run, and registered by the local authority. Discuss with your doctor or health visitor what arrangements exist in your area. If a private home is decided upon and is too expensive for you, the Department of Health and Social Security will advise you about whether you are entitled to financial assistance.

Financial support

Tax relief   Your relative will be considered your dependant and you are entitled to tax relief accordingly.

Pensions   Make sure your relative is receiving all the money he or she should. As well as the state pension, there may be a private pension scheme that is due and has been overlooked.

Disability grants   If your relative is registered as disabled or partially disabled, there will be money available for the necessary aids, for example, a wheelchair, walking aids, or a free radio for the blind. Contact the Disabled Living Foundation for advice (see below).

Home improvement   You should be eligible for grants towards the cost of adapting your home. Putting in a downstairs bathroom, or altering the existing one, improving insulation, making the electrical system safe and adequate with regard to lighting all come under this heading. Apply to the DHSS for information.

Heating grants are also available (these are important if your relative is still living alone and may be vulnerable to hypothermia – see Chapter 3. An increased allowance is given to the elderly during especially cold weather).

Travel   Old age pensioners travel free on local buses outside rush hours. A travel card is issued by the DHSS provided proof of eligibility (age) is shown.

Entertainment   Many local authorities allow OAPs free swimming at specified times, and cinemas often have a cheap day or, in some areas, only charge half price for OAPs. Museums and galleries usually reduce admission fees for pensioners.

USEFUL ADDRESSES

Age Concern
Bernard Sunley House
60 Pitcairn Road
Mitcham
Surrey CR4 3LL

Alzheimer's Disease Society
3rd Floor
Bank Buildings
Fulham Broadway
London SW6 1EP

Association to Aid the Sexual and Personal Relationships of the Disabled
286 Camden Road
London N7 0BJ

Association of Carers
Medway House
Balfour Road
Rochester
Kent ME4 6QU

British Red Cross Society
(*supplies nursing and mobility equipment at a low rent*)
9 Grosvenor Crescent
London SW1X 7EJ

Disabled Living Foundation
380–384 Harrow Road
London W9 2HU

Help the Aged
1 Sekforde Street
London EC1R 0BE

National Association for Carers and their Elderly Dependants
29 Chilworth Mews
London W2 3RG

North America: The United States

Medical help
Your family doctor or specialist in geriatrics can provide skilled care for your relative. He or she will arrange for admission to the hospital or a suitable nursing home in the event of serious illness.

Home nursing is organized through public and private hospitals and a variety of sponsoring agencies, usually under the physician's orders

You may ask for regular assistance with physical and speech therapy, with specialist nursing (applying dressings, giving injections) and with the heavy work of lifting and bathing. The personnel providing this assistance are trained nurses and specialist therapists. Expenses are normally met by Medicare, Medicaid for those over sixty-five, or by a private health insurance plan. Medicare covers certain prescribed costs deemed medically necessary but does *not* cover custodial – that is, routine, unskilled – care. Medicaid assistance is open to people on very low incomes (call your County Department of Social Services for information). Veterans Administration hospitals organize assistance for home health care in some areas. Also, the local Area Agency on Aging (with the federal-level Administration on Aging and the State Units on Aging) can help coordinate a comprehensive service-delivery system.

Hospice care
Medicare (Part A, Hospital Insurance) will cover care for a terminally ill person at home if the care is provided by a Medicare-certified hospice program.

Shared care

Day care clubs   These supply a lot of enjoyment and stimulation for an elderly person living with relatives. They are numerous nationwide though obviously more common where there is a large elderly population. For those on low incomes part of the expense may be met by Medicaid. Most are sponsored by religious, fraternal or community organizations or by a hospital clinic.

Respite care provides full time assistance while you are away, for example, during working hours. Information is available through the home health agencies and Area Agencies on Aging.

Vacations   There are also respite centers where a short stay can be arranged while you take your vacation. Try to make a careful assessment, together with your relative, of the homes in your area well in advance, and be sure there will be a vacancy in the one you choose. In the Sun Belt, there are hotels especially for guests over sixty-five and these are very popular for holidays with more active elderly people.

Financial support

Social security   This is a variable amount, fixed according to income and other factors. If your elderly relative is dependent on you for support, one-third of the maximum entitlement per month is deducted from the payment he or she would receive if self-supporting; you can take a deduction on your own income taxes in return. It is important to know the ins and outs of the system to be sure you are receiving your due. For information, write to the Social Security Administration, or consult *The Social Security Book* by Jack E. Gaumnitz (Arco Publishing, Inc., New York), which explains the Social Security system – including Medicare – in layman's terms, with case histories and advice on how to be sure you are given all the assistance you are entitled to.

Disability Large organizations such as the American Red Cross lend aids for the disabled (walking aids and so on) at low cost. Medication and expensive equipment such as wheelchairs or special beds come under health insurance (Medicare or private). Payments are allowed on case-by-case assessment.

Special benefits
Senior citizens are eligible for reduced travel fares and for reduced-rate tickets for theater and other entertainment.

If your relative lives in his or her own home, some assistance can be obtained on heating bills; certain property-tax reductions may also apply. Elderly people who sell their homes can exempt capital gains from the sale from their income taxes.

For information about these and other benefits, contact your Area Agency on Aging or other local agencies.

USEFUL ADDRESSES

Administration on Aging
Office of Human Development Services
US Dept of Health and Human Services
330 Independence Avenue, SW
Washington, DC 20201

American Association of Retired Persons
1909 K Street NW
Washington, DC 20049

American Association of Retired Persons
Western Office
Andrus Building
215 Long Beach Boulevard
Long Beach, CA 90801

American Hospital Association
Division of Ambulatory and Home Care Services

840 N Lake Shore Drive
Chicago, Il 60611

American Red Cross
National Headquarters
17th and D Streets
Washington, DC 20006

Council of Community Health Services
National League of Nursing
10 Columbus Circle
New York, NY 10019

Home Health Services and Staffing Association
2101 L Street, NW
Washington, DC 20037

National Association of Area Agencies on Aging
600 Maryland Avenue, SW
Suite 208
Washington, DC 20024

National Association of Home Care
205 C Street, NE
Washington, DC 20002

National Homecaring Council
67 Irving Place
New York, NY 10003

Social Security Administration
6401 Security Blvd
Baltimore, MD 21235

Canada

In British Columbia there is a Long Term Care Program open to all residents. Home care (nursing, physiotherapy etc) is provided free of charge where necessary and homemaker services (bathing, cleaning etc) to the needy. A contribution for this service is required from others according to their income. Meals on wheels, the Red Cross Loan Service and Rehabilitation are open to people in this program.

Day care centres, special treatment clinics for conditions such as arthritis, muscular dystrophy and mental illness, occupational therapy and mobile library services are organized by local communities. Medical

117

and hospital insurance is open to everyone who is a resident of British Columbia on payment of the premiums to the Medical Services Plan (see Useful Addresses). Pharmacare provides the elderly with prescription drugs free of charge.

Pensions The Canada Pension Plan is open to residents in all provinces except Quebec, but you must have joined during your working lifetime.

G.A.I.N. (Guaranteed Available Income for Need) is a monthly programme administered and funded by the Provincial Government for British Columbia residents who receive Federal Old Age Security Pension and Guaranteed Income Supplement.

USEFUL ADDRESSES

Capital Regional District Long-Term Care Administrator
Community Health Service
1947 Cook Street
Victoria, BC V8T 3B8

Vancouver Long-Term Care Administrator
Vancouver City Health Department
828 West 8th Avenue
Vancouver, BC V5Z 1E2

Social Planning and Review Council of British Columbia
(for further information)
2210 West 12th Avenue
Vancouver, BC V6K 2N6

National Advisory Council on Ageing
Jeanne Mance Building
Ottawa
Ontario

Australia and New Zealand

Medical help
All pensioners in Australia are entitled to free medical care, consultation with general practitioners and care within public hospitals. Drugs are available without cost, and eye and ear services are available free. Dental services are also now more freely available at no cost to pensioners. Geriatric medicine has developed in most centres of population and specialist advice is available to family doctors.

Housing for an elderly relative has been developed in the form of granny flats. These are prefabricated units with a bedroom, living room, kitchen and bathroom, which can be erected in the back garden of a family so that the elderly relative is independent but under some form of supervision. The granny flats can be bought outright or hired.

Nursing and shared care

The District Nursing Service is available in all areas and relatives who care for a dependent elderly person in the house are entitled to a domiciliary nursing care benefit, some financial assistance in the caring role. In some areas a linen service is available for incontinent elderly people living at home. A home help service is widely available. The cost is subsidized and to most pensioners it comes free. Meals on wheels is widespread. It too is subsidized, and the cost per meal is low.

Support groups for various disabilities are developing, and Alzheimer's disease, strokes and Parkinson's disease have very active support groups now functioning. Day centres and day hospitals are widespread and in most cases transport is available to take an elderly person to the centre.

Relative relief admissions are now on an organized basis, with appropriate funding, and beds are available in public hospital nursing homes and in non profit making hostels.

Finance

All Australians are entitled to an old age pension, with the exception of recent arrivals who have been sponsored by relatives living in Australia and elderly citizens who have major assets. Pensioners are entitled to various financial reliefs with house rates, telephone rental, car licence and travel costs. Public transport is at reduced fares and taxis are available at half price for pensioners.

Home modifications and provision of aids within the house can be obtained through a scheme called The Provision of Aids for Disabled Persons and this can provide simple aids as well as quite sophisticated equipment if necessary.

The various State Councils on the Ageing have networks of information and advice and documentation about all entitlements for the elderly in Australia.

Nursing home finance   In the event of a patient becoming beyond care at home and requiring nursing home care, the Commonwealth Government provides a nursing home benefit which covers most of the cost for the nursing home.

Council on the Ageing
34 Argyle Place
Millers Point
Sydney NSW 2000

Council on the Ageing
The Adelaide Lions Club
23–27 Coglin Street
Adelaide SA 5000

Council on the Ageing
1st Floor
Wallace Bishops Building
230 Edward Street
Brisbane Qld 4000

Council on the Ageing
2 St John's Avenue
New Town
Hobart Tas 7008

Council on the Ageing
PO Box 2476
Darwin NT 2239

Council on the Ageing
11 Freedman Road
Mount Lawley
Perth WA 6050

Council on the Ageing
The Hughes Community Centre
Hughes
Canberra ACT 2605

Victorian Coucil on the Ageing
449 Swanston Street
Melbourne Vic 3000

New Zealand

Auckland Old People's Welfare Council Inc
PO Box 7139
Auckland

Canterbury Old People's Council Inc
PO Box 2355
Christchurch

Otago Old People's Welfare Council Inc
PO Box 5355
Dunedin

Presbyterian Social Services Association
Aged Care Division
Private Bag CPO
Auckland

Presbyterian Social Services Association
Aged Care Division
PO Box 13171
Christchurch

Presbyterian Social Services Association
Aged Care Division
PO Box 374
Dunedin

Presbyterian Social Services Association
Aged Care Division
PO Box 27000
Wellington

ACKNOWLEDGMENTS

I am indebted to Mary Banks for careful editing, done with such skill and tact that I agreed with all her suggestions to make my book clear and readable.

1986   M. KEITH THOMPSON

The publishers would like to thank the following for their help in the preparation of this book:

For permission to reproduce photographs: Richard and Sally Greenhill (page 85); Susan Griggs Agency (page 53); Remploy Medical Products (pages 25, 46); Department of Medical Photography, Westminster Hospital Medical School (pages 45, 67 *right*).

For her advice and supervision of the exercise sequences (pages 52 and 58), Mrs Penny Copple, Director of EXTEND (Exercise Training for the Elderly and Disabled), Sheringham Norfolk.

The photographs on pages 24, 41, 43, 52, 56, 58, 59, 63, 64, 77, 82 were taken by Ray Moller, assisted by Liz Gedney. The modelling was by Vera and Alf Chaney, and Sarah Kirkwood. Props were kindly lent by Chester-care Ortho Aids, London NW3, Dorma Ltd, Manchester and The Reject Shop, London, W1.

The diagrams are by Kevin Marks. The information for the calcium table on page 48 is based on *The Composition of Foods* (McCance and Widdowson, HMSO).

INDEX

Page numbers in *italic* refer to the illustrations.

Other books in the Positive Health Guide series

OVERCOMING ARTHRITIS
A guide to coping with stiff or aching joints
Dr Frank Dudley Hart

BEAT HEART DISEASE!
A cardiologist explains how you can help your heart and enjoy a healthier life
Prof Risteard Mulcahy

MIGRAINE & HEADACHES
Understanding, avoiding and controlling the pain
Dr Marcia Wilkinson

EYES
Their problems and treatments
Michael Glasspool, FRCS

DIABETES
A practical new guide to healthy living
Dr Jim Anderson

THE DIABETICS' DIET BOOK
A new high-fibre eating programme
Dr Jim Mann and the Oxford Dietetic Group

THE DIABETICS' COOKBOOK
Delicious new recipes for entertaining and all the family
Roberta Longstaff, SRD, and Dr Jim Mann

THE DIABETICS' GET FIT BOOK
The complete home workout
Jacki Winter
Introduction by Dr Barbara Boucher

DR ANDERSON'S HCF DIET
The new high-fibre low cholesterol way to keep slim and healthy
Dr James Anderson

THE SALT-FREE DIET BOOK
An appetizing way to help reduce high blood pressure
Dr Graham MacGregor

DON'T FORGET FIBRE IN YOUR DIET
To help avoid many of our commonest diseases
Dr Denis Burkitt

STRESS AND RELAXATION
Self-help ways to cope with stress and relieve nervous tension, ulcers, insomnia, migraine and high blood pressure
Jane Madders

ANXIETY AND DEPRESSION
A practical guide to recovery
Prof Robert Priest

THE HIGH-FIBRE COOKBOOK
Recipes for good health
Pamela Westland
Introduction by Dr Denis Burkitt

HIGH BLOOD PRESSURE
What it means for you and how to control it
Dr Eoin O'Brien and
Prof Kevin O'Malley